THE BEST DIET BOOK

EVER

Praise for
THE BEST DIET BOOK EVER

This certainly is *The Best Diet Book Ever*, with superb storytelling and invaluable insights. It is really resonating for many of my patients, and the feedback I get is unique, like your book. I just ordered more copies for our office to always have on hand.

—*Dr. William Sellman, M.D., MBA*
University Healthcare Alliance / Stanford Hospital & Clinics

Losing 60 pounds gave me the confidence that I could succeed at anything. I've kept the weight off and kept winning tournaments. Dr. Parent is a master, and this book will help you to lose weight, feel more confident, and achieve your goals.

—*Cristie Kerr, U.S. Open and LPGA Champion,*
#1 in Rolex World Ranking of Women's Golf

Dr. Joe offers an easy-to-read, no-nonsense approach that opens us up to enjoy our food…and our lives. Great information and practical strategies—I highly recommend it!

—*Susan Piergeorge, MS, RDN,*
Author of "Boomer Be Well," Nutritional Expert

Let me sing the praises of Dr. Joe's book—an important and timely work in light of our national weight crisis. This really is the best diet book ever! Get it and you won't regret it!

—*Michael Bolton, multiple Grammy Award—winning*
singer and songwriter

THE BEST DIET BOOK

EVER

The Zen of Losing Weight

by Best-Selling Author

DR. JOSEPH PARENT

with Nancy Parent and Ken Zeiger

ZEN ARTS PRESS

Design by Megan Parent

Cataloging-in-Publication Data is on file
with the Library of Congress

ISBN 978-0-9728469-2-9

Printed in the United Stated of America
December 2015
First Edition

Dedicated to my teachers,
Chögyam Trungpa Rinpoche and
Vajra Regent Ösel Tendzin,
who showed me the nature of mind
and the path to freedom.

And to my family, my friends, my wife,
dearest companions on this
journey through life.

Table of Contents

Introduction

"Taking the first step on your journey means
it is already half accomplished."

—Zen Proverb

This book has no recipes or prescriptions for what to eat or what to avoid. It will teach you a positive way of thinking about how you approach dieting, and ultimately about how you treat yourself in all facets of life. It will show you how to use your mind in a constructive way, free from self-defeating, negative attitudes.

New diet programs get introduced every year. These systems tell you exactly what to eat, how to eat, and when to eat. Why do so many people still have trouble losing weight? And why do so many who lose weight have trouble keeping the pounds off? The number one New Year's resolution is to lose weight and get fit. Sadly, it's also the least successful!

Most people find dieting unpleasant and frustrating—a continual struggle. It's usually the combination of a restrictive diet plan and how people go about trying to put it into practice that makes losing weight difficult.

It doesn't have to be that way.

This book presents an alternative that really does work: *The Positive Choice Model*. Making positive, rewarding choices and setting small, attainable goals is more effective than the usual negative, self-punishing approach to losing weight.

This is a diet book unlike any other. It doesn't tell you to change what you eat; it shows you how to change your state of mind and your way of living. This book doesn't teach you how to cook your food, it teaches you how to cook your mind. In this book you'll find no recipes or menus, no restrictions or deprivations. No rules, just tools.

What makes this *The Best Diet Book Ever* is that it complements any reasonable weight-loss plan. Think of it as a meta-program that gives you the tools to put whatever plan you adopt, or create for yourself, into action with maximum effectiveness. It offers you time-tested mindful awareness techniques. These include exercises for working with thoughts and emotions, for settling and centering your body and mind, and for changing unhelpful habits.

No matter how good your diet plan is, if you don't know how to work with your mind and emotions, you can't overcome the obstacles you'll encounter in your weight-loss journey. Stress, emotional reactivity, giving in to temptations, cravings, and peer pressure—all these triggers can make starting and sticking to a diet program very difficult.

The Best Diet Book Ever offers you a different way of looking at and experiencing the process of losing weight and keeping it off. *The Positive Choice Model* provides you with the proper foundation for making your next attempt at dieting a success.

This book's subtitle is *The Zen of Losing Weight*. What does Zen have to do with dieting? Zen means "action with awareness," being completely in the present moment. Zen practices broaden the mind, engendering confidence, focus, and awareness, as well as energy, stamina, and peaceful equanimity. The more you cultivate the Zen qualities of presence and awareness, the easier it will be to achieve your dieting goals.

Although there is a progression through the book that takes you on your journey, each chapter stands alone as well. Feel free to go straight to the chapters that provide tools you need for taking less in, burning more up, and keeping on track.

The opening section, **Taking a Different Perspective,** invites you to look at the weight-loss process with an open mind, full self-acceptance, and newfound confidence.

Section 2, **The NINJA System™: Change Without Pain,** presents a simple but powerful technique for cultivating good habits—an indispensable tool that will allow you to accomplish all of your objectives. You'll learn the practice of Mindful Awareness, and develop a non-judgmental relationship with your own thoughts and emotions. You'll learn how to turn your mind into an ally instead of an enemy.

Section 3, **Taking Less In**, offers a comprehensive collection of practical methods that you can simply and easily introduce into your daily life. You'll learn how to avoid the *Three Too's*: eating too much, too fast, for too long. You'll be able to replace them with the *Three S's*: eating smaller portions, more slowly, and stopping earlier.

Section 4, **Challenges to Taking Less In: Watch Your S.T.E.P.**, deals with the obstacles everyone faces in keeping the discipline of a dieting program. You'll get helpful suggestions for handling Stress, Temptations, Emotions, and Personality issues. You'll learn methods that will support you in navigating the ups and downs that accompany the weight-loss journey.

Section 5, **Burning More Up**, explains the importance of balancing diet and exercise, and provides profound yet simple methods for improving your exercise habits.

The Best Diet Book Ever concludes with guidelines for the long-term maintenance of your weight-loss program in Section 6, **Keeping On Track In Dieting and In Life**. This stage often proves to be even more difficult than dropping the weight in the first place. In the last few chapters you'll learn how you can apply the principles and practices from this book to all aspects of your everyday life.

Taking a
Different Perspective

"The definition of insanity is hoping to get a different result by doing the same thing over and over again. We can't solve problems by using the same kind of thinking we used when we created them."

—Albert Einstein

Good as Gold

There once was a young girl who had a small clay statue, a family heirloom. She'd always wished that it were bright shiny gold instead of plain brown clay. When she was old enough to earn some money doing small jobs, she saved what she earned until she could afford her special project: she took the statue to a jewelry store to have it covered with gold.

Now it looked just the way she wanted, and people admired it. She felt very proud that she had a gold statue. However, the gold-plating didn't stick to the clay very well, and before long it began to flake off in spots. So she had it gold-plated again. Soon she found herself using all her time to earn money for maintaining the gold façade of her statue.

One day her grandparents returned from a journey of many years. The young girl was excited to show them how she had made the clay statue into a gold one. However, clay was showing through in a few spots, so she was also somewhat embarrassed.

Her grandmother smiled and held the statue lovingly. She moistened her handkerchief and gently rubbed at one of the spots. "Many years ago the statue must have fallen in the mud and become covered with clay. As a very young child, you wouldn't have known the difference. You forgot, and thought it was just a clay statue. But look here."

Where she had rubbed, a bright yellow color shone through.

"You never needed to put gold on to cover the clay. All you have to do is gently remove the clay and reveal the solid gold statue you've possessed all along."

You are the gold. That's your essence, your nature.

Everyone has the capacity to appreciate the simple joy of being alive. It is the delight you feel from the view of a spectacular sunset, the sound of a beautiful piece of music, or the smile of a loved one. It is an experience of natural richness.

One of the core principles of the Zen tradition is that human beings by nature are basically good. Believing in your basic goodness is the confidence that nothing is faulty in your make-up; nothing is lacking.

This perspective of richness is not all that common. Many people relate to dieting with a kind of "poverty mentality." How often have you felt like a failure after a slip or binge? That comes from the mistaken belief that in order to be who you *want* to be, you need to be something other than who you are.

When our experiences of fear and self-doubt accumulate, obscuring our connection with basic goodness, we feel the need to prove our worth. We think that the only cure for such feelings of inadequacy is to gold-plate ourselves into something better.

You don't struggle with losing or maintaining your weight because there is something fundamentally wrong with you.

The real causes are negative attitudes toward yourself, mistaken ideas about dieting, and unhelpful habits that have built up over time. They are the clay.

Gold-plating yourself, covering up aspects that make you feel self-conscious or embarrassed, isn't necessary. You just have to gently start removing the clay. That means adopting a more positive attitude toward yourself, exploring new perspectives on dieting, and undoing some of your unhelpful habits.

Remember that you are the gold that is *always* there, beneath the surface. When you exchange your "poverty mentality" for a "richness mentality," having a bad day won't undermine your self-worth. Even in the midst of struggle or discouragement, there can be a joyful moment that connects you to the heart of goodness, like rays of the sun breaking through dark clouds. Appreciating those moments can transform your outlook.

It's important to recognize the difference between your nature and your habits. Thinking of your actions as part of your nature—"That's just the way I am"—makes them feel unworkable and unchangeable. However, seeing things you do as habits—"That's something I seem to do a lot"—means that there is always the possibility of change.

When you recognize that basic goodness is your true nature, you open the door to experiencing unconditional confidence. You'll feel empowered to conquer the habits that have been holding you back, freeing you to accomplish your goals of losing weight and keeping it off.

It'll Be Different This Time

"Poor decisions are what make you gain weight and better ones are what make you lose it. Your brain will respond to the changes you make, better than you think. And so will your body."

—from an interview at the Mayo Clinic

You may have tried to diet and struggled to lose weight. Or you succeeded in losing weight, but couldn't keep it off. If so, you probably approached dieting from a poverty mentality: "What's wrong with me? How did I let myself get this heavy? Why can't I stick to a diet?" If you believe there is something wrong with you, you'll eventually sabotage your own efforts and fail.

I never had a chance. My mother told me I'd always be overweight because I had an eating problem. Whenever I dieted I knew that I'd blow it eventually, so at the slightest discouragement I gave up.

When we were children, we got the message that we should be punished if we misbehaved. If we feel badly about ourselves for being overweight, we're likely to regard dieting as a form of self-punishment. We decide to diet, but start as if we're entering a prison, with unpleasant restrictions imposed on us as the penance we deserve.

Traditional diets fit this approach all too well. They often include harsh "should" and "shouldn't" commands. You are told what, when, and how much you can eat, as well as what is "off limits." They assume that you are helpless to resist food or make good choices, so you need to submit yourself to a program that makes the decisions for you.

Some diets allow you days off the regimen, but then describe those as "cheat days." That just makes you feel guilty. And going back to the diet prison the next day is even more painful than before.

Eventually you begin to resent that you don't have control, that you're being punished, and that you're imprisoned. You'll also resent the diet if you're doing it to be attractive to others, rather than for yourself. Resentment eventually leads to rebellion, so you sabotage your efforts and abandon the diet.

I let myself slip on a Friday, tell myself I'll start over Monday, and have a "get-out-of-jail-free" card for the weekend. I escape from Diet Jail and head for Binge City!

You delight in your temporary freedom, but you either feel remorse and guilt (*Why did I do that? I can never stick to a diet!*), or dish out blame (*This is another lousy diet that doesn't work!*).

Because you felt bad about yourself for being overweight, you went on a diet as punishment. Being on the diet felt like prison, so you escaped. Now you feel bad about yourself because you quit, so you beat yourself up for being a failure. The only thing that makes you feel better is to eat. And then you need to diet again. It's a no-win merry-go-round. But it doesn't have to be that way.

Imprisonment or Empowerment?

It'll be different this time. That may be something you've heard (or said to yourself) before, but this time it can actually come true.

Why will it be different? Because this time you will be empowered to diet based on your personal preferences rather than having to follow rules and regulations. This time you get to choose. What, when, and how much you eat is completely up to you. No one is going to tell you what you can't do or what you must do. It is much more powerful and effective when you choose how you relate to food and exercise.

This is the *Positive Choice Model* for losing weight. This time you can take personal responsibility to make choices that match your intention. Because you see yourself as the gold rather than the clay, your choice of how to diet is a positive one. How you eat and exercise is based on confidence and strength of intention rather than fear or weakness of willpower. Making positive choices is fundamental to self-empowerment. The more success you have in making such choices, the more empowered you'll feel in challenging situations.

Taking responsibility is a positive choice. You choose to eat and exercise in a way that supports your intention to lose weight, rather than feeling you are being deprived as punishment for being overweight. When you see foods that aren't healthy or helpful for weight-loss, now you'll feel *empowered* to say, "I don't need that," instead of feeling *resentful* that, "I can't have that."

Moving forward on your weight-loss journey will be based on your *positive choice* to weigh less and be in better shape. It takes some effort at the beginning, but you'll see that the results are worth it, because *you are worth it!*

These Glasses Work Great for Me

What is the best weight-loss program for you?

Most diet books present one system that is supposed to work for everyone. They recommend changes in the way a person eats and exercises, fitting everybody into that program, as if that's the only way to do things right.

Imagine going to an eye doctor for new glasses. He sits you down in the examination chair, takes off the glasses he's wearing and hands them to you, saying: "These glasses work great for me. This is the prescription I give to every one of my patients."

How fast would you be out of that office? No one would want an eye doctor like that. You need your own prescription, not someone else's.

Some diet programs recommend scheduling small meals throughout the day; others favor three balanced meals and no snacks. Some people get bored and need variety; others do better with a set menu. One thing is certain: no one diet formula works for everyone.

"There doesn't seem to be any "right" diet, and there doesn't seem to be any evidence that one particular diet will work better with an individual's specific metabolism. There's no magic diet. We know that pretty much any [reasonable] diet will help you lose weight if you follow it."

—from an interview at the Mayo Clinic

Within the basic framework of eating less, eating healthier, and exercising more, individual differences determine what works best for each person.

Most diets tell you what to eat and not eat: high carb, low carb; high protein, low protein; high fat, low fat; lots of grains, no grains; lots of dairy, no dairy—the list goes on. And it seems to change regularly. Are coffee, wine, or chocolate good for you or bad for you? If you don't like the answer, check back in a few months.

The setting is the distant future. Two doctors are talking about a man revived from a frozen sleep of 200 years:

"Has he asked for anything special?"

"Yes. For breakfast he requested something called wheat germ, organic honey, and tiger's milk."

"Oh yes, those were the charmed substances that some years ago were felt to contain life-preserving properties."

"You mean there was no deep fat? No steak or cream pies or hot fudge?"

"Those were thought to be unhealthy. Precisely the opposite of what we now know to be true."

"Incredible!"

—from the sci-fi comedy film, *Sleeper*

9

Food fads come and go. That's why in this book you won't find any recipes or menus. Nor are there any lists of required or prohibited foods.

What you *will* find are explanations of the attitudes, skills, and strategies that can help you choose and practice your ideal diet regimen, the one that gives you the best opportunity for success.

What I love about this book is that I get to eat whatever I want! At the same time, it has helped me make choices to eat less, stop eating earlier, and skip some less healthy foods. And those simple, painless changes translated into shedding six pounds the first month.

First you need to decide that you're ready to make the commitment to start dieting. Reflect on your current eating and exercise habits. Your diet plan should reinforce what you're already doing well and provide alternatives to the habits you want to change. This book offers you the tools that will enable you to make those changes.

In using the techniques explained here, please remember that they are not etched in stone. Though the principles of how the mind and body function are universal, the ideal combination of methods for taking these insights and applying them are entirely unique to you. They offer you possibilities to explore as you embark on your personal weight-loss journey.

Please note: The advice of a qualified health professional should be sought before you begin any new diet, exercise, or other wellness program.

Empty Your Cup

A young man read all the books he could find about Zen. He heard about a great Zen master and requested an appointment with him to ask for teachings. When they were seated, the young man proceeded to tell the master everything he had understood from his reading.

After some time, the master suggested that they have tea. He performed the traditional tea ceremony while the student sat at attention, bowing when served, saying nothing. The master began to pour tea into the student's cup. He poured until it was full, and kept pouring. The tea ran over the edge of the cup and onto the table. The master kept pouring as the tea ran off the table and onto the floor. Finally, the student couldn't contain himself any longer. He shouted, "Stop! Stop pouring! The cup is full—no more will go in!"

The master stopped pouring and said, "Just like this cup, your mind is full of your own opinions and preconceptions. How can you learn anything unless you first empty your cup?"

You may have tried many different diets, and already have many fixed ideas about what works and what doesn't. If your mind is closed, if you're not open to trying something new, your cup is full.

The empty cup approach doesn't mean giving up your intelligence and following blindly. The point is to receive everything that's presented in an open way, withholding judgment until you've looked a little deeper. Try your best to understand what is being communicated, then give it a fair chance to see whether it works for you.

Before starting a new weight-loss program, look at the assumptions about dieting that you may have carried with you for a while. Don't automatically buy into the latest information from the web that tells you what's good or bad for you. In computer lingo, you need to "empty your cache."

Shunryu Suzuki Roshi, a great Zen master, said, "In the beginner's mind there are many possibilities; in the expert's mind there are few." Beginner's mind is empty of preconceptions. It is inquisitive, receptive to whatever arises, and ready to engage.

No matter how much information you've collected about dieting, you can always take a fresh start and return to beginner's mind.

Think Outside the Lunchbox

"The exercises I do most regularly are
skipping the facts and jumping to conclusions."
—Diet Humor

We put information about people we know and things we experience into mental boxes that help us make sense of a very complex world. There is so much information out there, that to hold all of it at once is impossible. Based on past experience, our brain filters out certain things and files the rest into the appropriate categories.

Like emptying your cup, it's important to think outside your "dieting box." You may assume that dieting takes extraordinary willpower and requires a lot of self-punishment and deprivation. You may believe that you are unable to lose weight; that diets just don't work for you. But all of that isn't necessarily true. Recognize the assumptions you've made and let go of the misconceptions that are holding you back. Be open to the possibility that the experience of dieting could be something completely different.

The first step in your weight-loss journey is dropping (or at least suspending) all the negative ideas you have about dieting. Instead, approach it as a positive choice.

The origin of the word "diet" comes from the Greek *diaita* which means "a way of life." Thinking outside the box opens the door to embracing a new attitude toward eating, a new way of life that will help you achieve your weight-loss goals.

A Glimpse of the Future

If we truly want to be healthy and feel good, why is it so difficult to make the changes that will move us in that direction?

To make a positive choice to change your habits and lose weight, you need to have a strong desire and intention to do so. The problem is, it takes time to experience the benefits from dieting. You won't see a lower number on the scale or fit into a smaller size overnight. That means putting in the effort now, and not getting rewarded for it until later. Easy to say, but when you face temptation, immediate satisfaction usually wins out.

The target number on the scale seems far away and perhaps unrealistic. Doing it for your health is a nice idea, but it's easy to rationalize away.

How do I know I'll feel better? Even if I lose weight I could still get sick. I could get hit by a bus. I'm going to die someday anyway, why not go out with a belly full of chocolate ice cream?

Just hearing how much better you'll feel won't be enough. No matter how much anyone tells you dieting is good for you— that you'll look and feel better—those are all just words that sound like a lot of "Blah, blah, blah…"

What you need is a demonstration that will prove to you that the effort to start a weight-loss journey and change your habits is worth it. Words won't convince you, only experiences will convince you. Promises of a better future can't match the comforting feeling that food gives you *now*, especially if you are eating to soothe your stress, depression, or boredom. It's just hard to imagine being lighter and thinner.

Here's the good news: you can actually *feel* how much better it will be to weigh less, in advance! There's a way to have a glimpse of the future, a bridge from where you are to where you could be.

The Weigh-Less exercise will let you experience what it will actually feel like to weigh less and be slimmer. That feeling will reinforce your intention to lose weight. It will inspire you to overcome inertia and take action.

Weigh-Less Exercise

Want to immediately experience how good you'll feel when you are literally lighter on your feet?

Put ten to fifteen pounds of groceries in a shopping bag. [**Please note:** How heavy a bagful you choose depends on your weight. Please be careful not to use more than 10% of what you weigh, and no more than 20 pounds.]

Sit on the front edge of a stable (not rolling) chair and hold the bag against your stomach. Then stand up and feel how hard you have to work. Repeat three times.

Next, put the bag aside and stand up without the extra weight.

Feel how much easier it is, how good it feels with less weight on your legs and knees. Now you know—maybe your legs aren't so weak and your knees aren't so bad. Maybe they're just overworked!

Next, carefully pick up the bag and walk around for a minute or two. (You can climb a few stairs as long as you don't strain yourself.) That's what it will feel like if you put on those extra pounds. So if you're not sure you're ready to start *losing* weight, this might at least inspire you to make the changes that will prevent you from *gaining* weight.

The Weigh-Less exercise is the direct experience of feeling lighter, encouraging you to make the positive healthy choices of eating less and eating better.

I did the Weigh-Less exercise by walking around carrying two of my husband's 10-pound dumbbells (that's how much weight I wanted to lose). I thought I was in pretty good shape, but in no time my heart was pounding. What a load I've been putting on my system! Knowing how that felt made it much easier to opt for smaller portions and to skip dessert.

You'll be reminded to do the Weigh-Less exercise throughout this book. It's an important motivator that will inspire you to:

- Start the weight-loss journey without delay,
- Keep going through periods of no-change or discouragement, and
- Maintain your weight once you've reached your target.

Excess Baggage

The all-time highest rated episode of The Oprah Winfrey Show began with Oprah announcing, "I've lost 67 pounds, and fit into my size-10 Calvin Klein jeans again for the first time in seven years."

She went off-stage for a moment, and came back wheeling a red wagon with a big plastic bag of fat sitting on it.

She continued, "For those of you who are starting dieting — this is what 67 pounds of fat looks like! I can't lift it! Is this gross, or what? It is amazing to me that I can't lift it, but I used to carry it around with me every day! My poor heart!"

Airlines charge a fee for extra baggage that puts stress on a plane. The harder a plane has to work, the sooner it breaks down and needs to be repaired.

We should look at our bodies the same way—the more weight we carry, the harder we have to work, and the more likely we'll suffer physical breakdowns. One expression of being kind to yourself is putting less burden on your knees, feet, hips, and back.

Every calorie you consume but don't burn off will come at a price. Conversely, every pound you lose means more energy, less pain, and better overall health. This is part of the *Positive Choice Model*: choosing to eat less = weighing less = feeling less pain. This is a twist on a common sports motto: instead of "no pain, no gain," staying with your diet commitment means "no gain, no pain!"

Most people will gain about one pound for every 3500 calories they take in but don't burn off over a given period of time. If you usually eat two 450-calorie muffins a week, you can simply do without them and you will lose (or avoid gaining) a pound a month, or 12 pounds in a year! That's a serious extra baggage fee you save by foregoing a few muffins.

Reflect on recent experiences of body aches or tight-fitting clothes, and include relief from those as part of your positive choice equation. Is it worth the ongoing pain of carrying excess baggage for the temporary pleasure of eating more food? Or would you rather eat less and feel lighter? If you're in doubt, perform the Weigh-Less exercise to convince yourself.

Be Kind to Yourself

"Loving-kindness isn't about trying to throw ourselves away and become someone better. It's about befriending who we are already."

—Pema Chödrön, *Start Where You Are*

It's very easy to feel that dieting is a form of self-punishment. One reason is a message we've grown up with: we need to give ourselves a hard time if we make a mistake. However, research shows that negative feedback, from others or ourselves, only reinforces and strengthens the habits that we want to erase. The more we beat ourselves up for going on a binge, the more the thought of failure will be in our minds, and the easier it will be to give up and fall back into old patterns.

Feelings and attitudes give rise to thoughts and actions that become habits. To change your eating habits you have to change how you feel about yourself, including your attitudes toward eating and exercise. Instead of giving yourself a hard time when you have a setback, make the positive choice to be kind to yourself.

The Zen tradition talks about having an attitude of *maitri* (pronounced 'my-tree'), a Sanskrit word translated as "loving-kindness." The original meaning is the wish for everyone to be happy. But maitri also means making friends with yourself. It is the recognition of basic goodness as your true nature.

Within that, you can acknowedge both your confusion and your sanity without harsh judgment. This is a complete and radical acceptance of yourself, just as you are. A simple, direct relationship with how you feel and what you do is the expression of unconditional friendliness.

It's easy to confuse indulging yourself and truly being kind. Soothing your pain with a big helping of comfort food every time you are stressed isn't really kind. It's like giving a child candy every time they pester you for it—they are happy for a little while, then they get a stomach ache. When you really need nourishment for your spirit, filling your stomach isn't the answer. You'll feel good for a little while, and then feel bad later when you get on the scale.

If your goal is to stay with your weight-loss program, make the choices that will help you do so. Being kind to yourself means being your own best friend. Take the supportive attitude toward yourself that a good friend would:

- Encourage yourself to stick with your program.
- Remind yourself of your intention when you waver.
- Forgive yourself when you slip.

A friend of mine was upset that she had overeaten at a fancy dinner, and was putting herself down and calling herself names. I said, "Hey, don't talk about my friend like that! She doesn't deserve it! She may have made a mistake, but she's a good person!"

Introduction to Maitri Practice

Begin by sitting comfortably, in a good upright posture. Good posture makes it easier to breathe fully and stay attentive. Gently close your eyes and relax any tension you're feeling.

Move your awareness to the center of your body at heart level. Say to yourself, "My nature is the gold of basic goodness, and I deserve peace and happiness."

Tune in to any negative feelings about yourself—angry, sad, tired, and so on. Notice where you feel them in your body.

Imagine that, as you breathe in, you gather the negative feelings from all around your body into your heart center where they dissolve.

Like an air conditioner turning hot, sticky air into a cool, light breeze, the negative emotions transform into peace and contentment.

As you breathe out, radiate that peace and happiness from your heart center to all areas of your body.

Repeat this sequence with each in- and out-breath for a few minutes. Conclude by saying, "I feel the peace and happiness that I deserve. May others also feel the peace and happiness they deserve."

[**Please note:** Persons with respiratory issues should consult a health professional before doing any breathing exercise.]

Unconditional Confidence

"Confidence is an attitude that makes the seemingly unworkable workable. This doesn't mean that all of a sudden everything is going to go our way. But it does mean that we can appreciate life even when things don't go our way. We have the resources to live in the challenge. That is the expression of courage."

—Venerable Chögyam Trungpa,
Shambhala: The Sacred Path of the Warrior

Unconditional confidence is rooted in basic goodness and maitri. You believe in and are kind to yourself, even if you've strayed from your diet program in some way. You have the choice of identifying with the gold of your nature or the clay of your habits. You could dwell in the poverty mentality of feeling you are a hopeless case who is a failure at dieting, or see yourself as a successful dieter who has overeaten on occasion. It's up to you. As the old saying goes: "Believe you can or believe you can't, either way you're right."

When you have an attitude of unconditional confidence, day-to-day challenges won't determine how you feel about yourself. You may not be able to control what happens to you, but you can decide how you will respond. You can find a way to put anything in a positive perspective.

Unconditional confidence means trusting in your self-worth and capabilities, regardless of how things have been going lately. Reflect on the times you've eaten well, exercised regularly, and overcome challenges to your program. The better you feel about yourself, the better you can weather the ups and downs you'll encounter during the course of your weight-loss journey.

POINTS TO REMEMBER
FROM PART 1

- Perspective of basic goodness
  - Richness, not poverty
  - Identify with your nature, not your habits
- Choose a plan that's right for you
- Empty your cup and think outside the box
- Positive Choice Model:
  - Dieting as choice, not punishment
  - Empowered, not imprisoned
- Weigh-Less Exercise
- Be your own best friend
- Attitude of unconditional confidence

2

The NINJA System™
Change Without Pain

"As the thinking mind begins to settle through the practice of meditation, we start to see our patterns and habits far more clearly. When we apply the instruction to be soft and non-judgmental to whatever we see, there's room for genuine inquisitiveness. Each moment is an opportunity to make a fresh start."

—Pema Chödrön

Time to Choose

"Between every stimulus and response there is a space. In that space is our power to choose our response. In our response lies our growth and our freedom."

—Viktor E. Frankl, *Man's Search for Meaning*

The *Positive Choice Model* is the best approach to dieting because having the freedom to choose is better than being imprisoned by punishing restrictions. Having a side salad with your hamburger instead of fries is a positive choice *if* you want to skip the French fries as part of your weight-loss program. But denying yourself and feeling like it's a punishment to eat the salad will not only make you unhappy, it will also add pressure on your psyche that could lead to a future binge of fried-food madness.

To make a choice, there has to be the space and time to do so. Usually there's an automatic reaction from thought to eating. It happens so fast that the food is in your mouth before you know it. There is no awareness of how it happened.

There needs to be time to be aware of what's going on, and space to respond rather than react. Such decision points are like forks in the road. When you're speeding along you may miss your turn, and find yourself heading the wrong way.

Impulse arises ➔ reactively eat.

Impulse arises ➔ awareness ➔ choice to eat or not.

Without awareness of a decision point there is no option: when the impulse arises, you reactively eat.

With awareness, when the impulse arises, you have the choice to either eat or say, "No, thank you."

Reflect on your intentions for dieting. Remember the Weigh-Less exercise, and that you prefer the feeling of being lighter to the temporary satisfaction of eating.

When you opt not to eat, it's a positive choice, not a restriction or punishment. To be able to make that choice, you need time and space for awareness. The goal is to experience that awareness as much as possible.

You Must Be Present to Win

"YOU MUST BE PRESENT TO WIN" is often printed on a raffle ticket, but it has a deeper meaning here. To succeed in your weight-loss program, to make better choices, your mind and body need to be synchronized. That can only happen in the present, in the here and now.

Your body is always "here," and only exists "now." However, like everyone, your mind often strays, re-playing past events or projecting into the future. You have to practice bringing your attention back to the "here and now" when it wanders.

In the Zen tradition, this one-pointed attention is called *mindfulness* because your mind is full of the experience of the present moment. Mindfulness is being precisely focused on what your body and mind are doing, whether you are sitting still or in motion. It is sometimes referred to as *bare attention*, or *just noticing*. You experience each moment without adding anything to it mentally. You simply notice what appears in your mind without judging, categorizing, or commenting on it.

Mindfulness takes place in the atmosphere of *awareness*, the environment within which your thoughts and perceptions come and go, moment by moment. With precision and perspective, you can be mindfully aware of your world and yourself, constantly present and responsive to whatever arises.

Awareness includes noticing when you're off in a daydream and when you've returned to wakefulness. If your mind is wandering in distraction, you aren't bringing your full attention to what you're doing. That's why "you must be present to win."

If we're always in the present, how do we learn from the past or plan for the future? Within the context of mindfulness, it's fine to think about something in the past or the future. The key is to be aware that you are reflecting or planning, but that you are doing so within the present moment.

You can have thoughts of the past or future, understanding that they are just thoughts. You are aware of them, but aren't letting your attention be swept away by them.

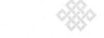

Know Your Mind

"Thoughts are to the mind as clouds are to the sky."
—Zen Proverb

Like the saying, "Seeing is believing," we often take the attitude, "Thinking is believing." When we have thoughts about ourselves or others, we take them to be true and instantly react to them, often producing painful results. Our thoughts are controlling us, rather than the other way around.

How can we free ourselves from the tyranny of our own thoughts? The insight leading to that freedom comes from asking another question: "Who or what is watching our thoughts?" Since it isn't someone else watching our thoughts, it must be our own mind.

When we look closely, we discover that the nature of mind is pure, content-free awareness. A clear glass jar takes on the color of whatever fills it. In the same way, mind is clear awareness that takes on the colors and textures of our thoughts and emotions. This nature of mind can only be discovered by direct examination through the practice of mindful awareness.

You have thoughts, but you are not your thoughts. The way to practice is to recognize unhelpful thoughts and hear them— but not listen to them! Just because you think, "I'll have a little more," doesn't mean you have to do it.

The Nature of Change

If you wanted to make a flower blossom, would you pull up on the stem? Or peel back the leaves to force it open? If you tried to make it blossom that way, you might actually kill it.

You can't make a flower blossom; you can only foster what it does naturally. If you give it the right conditions—sunlight, water, and good soil—the flower will blossom beautifully on its own. A flower doesn't *try* to blossom, it just does. That's its nature.

In the same way, as human beings it's our nature to grow and flourish. As a child, you didn't have to try to grow taller. With the right nourishment and environment, it happened.

You don't need to force yourself to develop your abilities. It's your nature to do so. All you need to do is give yourself the right conditions. They include the pure water of your inherent basic goodness, the warm sunlight of maitri, the rich soil of unconditional confidence and necessary intentions, the fresh air of non-judgmental awareness, and the fertilizer of knowledge and practice. With these in your environment, your natural tendencies to learn and grow will blossom.

Change Without Pain

A young monk was spending some time each day in meditation and contemplation. He wondered how many of his thoughts during those sessions were positive (about being generous, kind, or helpful) or negative (expressing prejudice, greed, or hatred toward others or himself). He collected a pile of pebbles and placed an empty bowl on each side, one labeled "positive" and the other "negative."

As he meditated, he would put a pebble in the appropriate bowl when he recognized either a positive or negative thought. At the end of the first day he looked down to see how he had done, and was surprised to see that all the pebbles were in the "negative" bowl.

Without judging himself, he simply continued this practice, starting over each day. After a few days, the number of pebbles in the two bowls was about equal. After a few more days, almost all the pebbles were in the "positive" bowl.

The NINJA System™ stands for the initials of the words "Necessary Intention & Non-Judgmental Awareness." To overcome an undesirable habit, first it's *necessary* to establish a strong *intention* to make a change. You then need to apply *non-judgmental awareness* to the unwanted actions, words, or thoughts. Each time you become aware of a habit that you intend to change, you record it—without judgment. A detailed explanation of that process follows this chapter.

Like a flower blossoming naturally, by just noticing, without adding judgments of good or bad, you'll find that you catch yourself sooner and sooner. At first you only notice what you did after it happened. Then you realize it *while* it's happening. After that you catch it just as it starts. Eventually you become aware of the impulse that drives the habit, and at some point even the impulse no longer appears. The habit is gone.

Your habits change because of the combination of intention and awareness. If your choice is to weigh less, you'll feel out of sync when your actions don't match your intention. To make changes, first you have to recognize what's getting in the way of your dieting objectives. If you don't know what's in the way, how do you know what to change?

You not only need to abandon and refrain from unhelpful habits like eating in front of the television or snacking late at night; you also need to cultivate and nurture helpful habits like eating slowly and mindfully and exercising regularly. Both building and dismantling habits require mindful awareness of your thoughts and actions.

The NINJA System is a powerful method for implementing the *Positive Choice Model*, the approach of personal preference rather than imposed restrictions. You are empowered to choose the way you would prefer to act, speak, or think, and then move in that direction. To judge, punish, or deprive yourself is counter-productive.

The old motto, "If at first you don't succeed, try, try again," is only true if you know the right way to try. Unfortunately, the way most people go about trying harder at dieting usually takes them farther from their goals. If you recognize that it is your nature to learn and grow, you can trust yourself to create the optimum conditions for success.

The following four questions, adapted from Dr. William Glasser's *Reality Therapy*, will help you clarify your objectives:

1. What do you want to accomplish?

   (Example: Losing 10 pounds)

2. What have you been doing that has helped you accomplish it?

   (Example: Walking for 20 minutes each day)

3. What have you been doing that has kept you from accomplishing it?

   (Example: Having a high-calorie snack before bed every night)

4. If you're not accomplishing what you want, what could you do differently?

   (Example: Erase the late-night snacking habit)

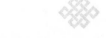

Applying *NINJA*

It's tempting whenever we start something new to do too much, too fast. We want it all and we want it now! You'll probably think of a list of habits you want to start changing right away. Trying to change too many at once doesn't work well.

Choose one or two at most. When a negative habit is erased, or a positive habit has become second nature, only then should you start working on the next one. As it says in the old fable, "Slow and steady wins the race."

There are different ways to apply *The NINJA System* for changing habits. You'll need a *"NINJA* Notepad"—a page on your phone or tablet, or a paper pad or index card.

Are you ready?

Make a Tally Mark

Write a key word or phrase on your notepad, and put a tally mark next to it each time you repeat either a negative or positive habit. Habits you want to erase may include "going back for seconds," "stopping at a fast food drive-thru," or "eating food straight from the container." Habits you want to develop may include "drinking water instead of snacking," "sharing an entrée," or "put food away before you start eating."

PUT EXTRA FOOD AWAY BEFORE EATING

﹋ﾄﾄﾄﾄﾄ I

Count the marks at the end of the day without judging how you did, just re-establishing your intention to change. Many people see the daily total shift dramatically in a relatively short period of time—more marks for positive habits, less marks for negative habits.

Another way of making a tally mark is to use letters and/or symbols. For example, you may want to erase the habit of eating when you are bored and replace it with a healthier activity. Write BOREDOM EATING on your notepad. Mark down a "B" each time you realize you are eating out of boredom; mark down an "R" each time you replace boredom eating with something like stretching or going for a walk.

Rate from Zero-to-Five

There are habits you'll want to change that are not "all or nothing," but instead appear in degrees. It works best to rate these on a scale of zero-to-five (representing the minimum and maximum amount the habit appears).

As an example of how to cultivate a helpful habit using a rating scale, let's say you want to slow down your eating speed After each meal, rate the speed at which you felt you just ate, where $0 =$ slow and mindful, and $5 =$ wolfing your food. Gradually you'll see more and more ratings of 1 or 0, meaning that you have successfully ingrained the habit of eating slowly and mindfully.

EATING SPEED

Day 1:breakfat 5/ lunch3/dinner 3

Day 2: breakfast 4/ lunch 2/ dinner 2

Day 3: breakfast 2/ lunch 1/ dinner 1

The *NINJA System* can help you change the way you eat, as well as how you act, how you speak, and even how you think. You can create routines that erase negative habits and make positive habits second-nature. You'll feel empowered to get out of your own way and get the most out of your capabilities.

NINJA Your Food Thoughts:

Emily was the kind of person who "lives to eat" rather than "eats to live."

It's hard for me to imagine that there are people who are not thinking about food most of the time. I can't believe when someone says they forgot to eat a meal. If I'm not thinking about food, what else would I be thinking about?

Emily wrote the words THINKING ABOUT FOOD on her notepad. Each time she found herself lost in thought about eating, she made a mark. She did her best not to judge herself, but to just keep count. She thought about food less and less often as the days passed, and her eating thoughts were replaced by positive thoughts about people to call, places to go, and things to do.

Write It Down

You can use *The NINJA System* in support of your weight-loss program by keeping a log of your eating and exercise choices.

A glass of water or two donuts? A half-hour in front of the television or a brisk walk? Knowing that you'll be accountable after each meal and exercise session increases awareness of your intentions and actions. The choices are yours; logging them will move you toward making better ones.

You can also give yourself a zero-to-five rating after each meal, noting how much more or less you ate than you had planned. Reflect on your *Necessary Intention* and notice with *Non-Judgmental Awareness* how you did.

It's important not to judge or punish yourself when you make your entries; otherwise you might avoid logging because you feel guilty about what or how much you ate.

Writing it down allows you to be aware of everything you've eaten up to that point in the day. That way you can make informed positive choices for your next meal that match your intention.

You can think of *The NINJA System* as a sort of written contract with yourself to eat less, eat healthier, and exercise more.

Try This:

Practice recording what and how much you're planning to eat in your log *before* each meal. It's easier to be mindful when you have a plan. It provides a boundary that helps you choose the appropriate portion size as you prepare and serve the meal. Knowing that you'll have to write it down if you eat more than you intended strengthens your resolve to stick to your plan.

Necessary Intention

Question: How many psychologists
does it take to change a light bulb?
Answer: Only one, but the light bulb
has to really want *to change.*

—Psychologist Humor

There's often truth in humor—when it comes to your eating and exercise habits: to make a change you have to really *want* to change. That is Necessary Intention.

There is inertia in human behavior, just as there is in the physical world. Inertia means that a body at rest tends to stay at rest (unless moved), while a body in motion tends to stay in motion (unless blocked). It's hard to get off that couch, but once you've made the effort to get up and move, it's not so hard to keep moving. It's hard to stop moving when you have been busy, but when you've made the effort to sit down and practice mindful awareness, it's not hard to stay there a while.

It takes effort to make that first positive step over the threshold of inertia. That's why changing habits requires the strength of Necessary Intention to get you moving, and Non-Judgmental Awareness to keep you on track.

To maintain and reinforce your motivation during lulls or plateaus as you progress in your journey, it's helpful to repeat the Weigh-Less exercise. It reminds you how good it will feel if you stay with the program and get lighter. That fires up your Necessary Intention to keep tracking your progress with Non-Judgmental Awareness.

NINJA *your Weigh-Less Exercise:*

Develop the habit of doing the Weigh-Less exercise on a regular basis. On your calendar, mark " WL" each day that you do the Weigh-Less exercise. That will help you to reflect on your Necessary Intention during decision points at meal times. Is the food you're about to eat worth the calories, or would you rather feel lighter and thinner? The choice is up to you, without judgment about which you choose.

The Power of Commitment

A councilman asked an old farmer to be part of a citizens committee that would work to improve various things about the town. The farmer asked, "Do you want me to be involved or committed?"

Puzzled, the man asked, "What's the difference?"

The farmer answered, "It's like a bacon and eggs breakfast. The chicken is involved, but the pig is committed."

Commitment is the backbone of Necessary Intention. It supports the continuity of your efforts over time and across situations. Commitment means putting your heart into the dieting and exercise plans you've made for enhancing wellness in your life.

To be able to commit to a plan, you need to feel that you can handle any outcome—you need to be willing to pre-accept whatever the results might be. After a slip, a binge, or in the periods of time when it seems like you're not making progress, it's crucial to stay committed to your weight-loss program.

Having commitment doesn't guarantee perfect results, but it will give you the best chance of achieving your goals. On the occasions that you fall short or have a setback, you can give yourself a break and recharge your aspiration, intention, and commitment. Getting frustrated and giving yourself a hard time for being less than perfect is discouraging, making it more likely that you'll give up.

Be 100 percent optimistic and committed to your program before you start, and then 100 percent realistic (and forgiving and kind to yourself!) about the ups and downs along the way.

Keep Your Scale in the Kitchen

"Keep your scale in the kitchen—
you won't eat as much if you know it's watching you."
—Diet Humor

It's a joke, but go ahead and really do that if it supports your commitment. Use whatever will remind you of your Necessary

Intention to take less in. Maybe it'll "tip the scales" in favor of making positive choices such as taking smaller portions, selecting healthier options, skipping snacks, and eating more slowly. If you don't want to relocate your scale, you can put a picture of one on the fridge or food cabinet. Or put up a photo of a piece of clothing you'd like to fit into.

The point is to use something that will catch your eye and create a gap—the space and time for mindful awareness. Reinforcing your commitment keeps you from reacting mindlessly to an urge to splurge on an unplanned snack.

Try this:

Use sticky notes posted in key places around the house and at work with positive choice reminders written on them.

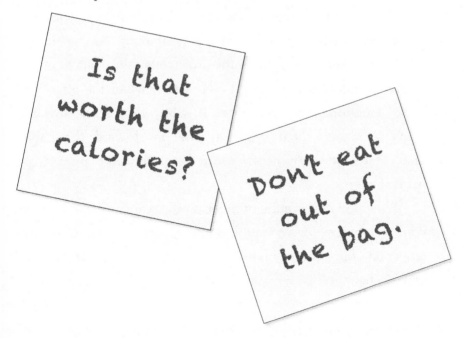

Non-Judgmental Awareness

"It is only when we begin to relax and relate with ourselves without moralizing, harshness, or deception that we can begin to let go of harmful patterns."

—Pema Chödrön

Whatever habit you're working on, hold it in the gentle space of Non-Judgmental Awareness. Be an objective observer of your own actions. This is different from self-consciousness, when you watch what you're doing with a critical eye, judging every experience.

It is generally accepted in psychology that *all* emotionally loaded attention, good or bad, is reinforcing. Any criticism, nagging, or anger you direct toward habits you want to erase actually reinforces those habits. However, when the attention is not emotional or judgmental, it subtly moves one toward whatever deeply held intention one has toward the habit. That is why Non-Judgmental Awareness is crucial to producing habit change.

When you observe the number on the scale or the entries in your weight-loss log without judgment, you can unemotionally reflect on your actions, rekindle your intentions, and resolve to make better choices.

Don't Be Afraid of Your Scale

"A little girl invited her friend to visit, and was showing her around the house. When they got to the bathroom, the little girl pointed to the scale and said, 'Don't go near that. It makes my mommy cry.'"

—Diet Humor

In the *Positive Choice Model*, the scale is your friend. When the number is going up, it motivates you to put more effort into eating well and exercising. When the number is going down, it is confirmation that your effort is paying off. Knowing you'll be recording the number, that you'll be accountable, reminds you of your Necessary Intention in challenging situations.

Success in a weight-loss program is usually determined by the number on the scale. Unfortunately, all too often that number is treated by a dieter as an indicator of his or her self-worth. Gain a pound and "I was bad this week," lose a pound and "I was good, but could have been even better."

When I'm "bad" it's not a little mistake; it's a catastrophe — I'm a failure, so why bother trying anymore?

The key is to relate to the number on the scale with Non-Judgmental Awareness. Don't use the number on the scale as a reason to beat yourself up. That undermines your intention.

When there is judgment involved, it brings emotion with it. Emotion clouds insight—you lose track of your intention and awareness of your actions. You can't think straight about your diet plan when you are emotionally bent out of shape.

Judging and criticizing yourself can reinforce unwanted habits and block your progress, sometimes to the point of sending you off on a binge, or even abandoning your program altogether. Keep the perspective of Non-Judgmental Awareness: the number is just a number—not an indictment of yourself and your capabilities.

NINJA your Attitude Toward the Weigh-In:

Use *The NINJA System* not just to track your weight, but also to change the habit of judging yourself. Rate from zero-to-five to indicate how much you BEAT YOURSELF UP after you see the number on the scale. You'll gradually be kinder to yourself and more patient with your progress.

Here's an example of the ratings of someone who weighed herself every Monday and Thursday:

WEIGH-INS
140; 142; 141; 140; 139; 140; 139; 141; 140; 139

BEATING MYSELF UP AFTER WEIGHING IN
3; 5; 4; 3; 1; 2; 0; 1; 0; 0

It's important to weigh yourself on a regular basis—once or twice a week, every day, or every other day—the interval doesn't matter as much as keeping up the schedule. For consistency, weigh yourself at the same time of day, wearing the same amount of clothes (or lack of clothes). Don't worry if you miss a weigh-in here or there. Just not too many in a row, and don't skip because you're afraid of what the scale will say.

I weigh myself every morning before getting dressed and having breakfast. If it's higher than the day before, I reflect on what happened yesterday that might have caused that, such as eating (or drinking) too much or too late in the evening. If it's lower than the day before, it's a nice reward for staying on my program and an inspiration to maintain commitment to my weight-loss intention throughout the day.

Good to Know:

If part of your program includes significant muscle-building, the numbers on the scale may not be an accurate reflection of progress. Your physical condition and appearance will be better measures.

Helpful Hint:

If you are recording your ratings on a mobile device or computer, don't use negative emojis. They are images expressing negative emotions. Just notice and make your rating. A "frowny face" ☹ is the opposite of Non-Judgmental Awareness.

Practicing Mindful Awareness

Just as you need to work out on a regular basis to develop and sustain your physical fitness, you also need to strengthen your "mental muscles." You need to train your mind through the practice of mindful awareness.

You are training in order to:

- Pay better attention to what you are doing.
- Maintain that attention for longer periods of time.
- Notice more quickly when your attention wanders.
- Return more sharply to the here and now.

This chapter presents brief summaries of each phase of the practice. For fully detailed instructions, please turn to the Appendix.

Take Your Seat

Find a place where you can sit uninterrupted for as long as you intend to practice. For a beginner, it is helpful to find a quiet place, and practice for short periods of time.

While this is traditionally done sitting cross-legged on a cushion, most people find it easier to sit on a chair or footstool. If you use a chair, sit in the center of the seat without leaning against the back. It's helpful to have your knees level with or lower than your hips, to prevent strain on your legs and back. Your feet can be flat on the floor, or loosely crossed in front of you.

Good posture makes it easier to stay attentive, and easier to breathe. You'll want your spine to be upright but not strained. Imagine that your spine is like a tent pole and the rest of your body is the canvas hanging loosely from the top of the pole.

Let your arms hang straight down from your shoulders. Place your hands palms down, on top of each thigh just behind your knees; or palms up, one upon the other, in your lap.

Phases of Mindful Awareness Practice

[**Please note:** Persons with respiratory issues should consult a health professional before doing any breathing exercise.]

Phase 1: Grounding

Gently close your eyes. Let any excess tension, other than what you need to hold your posture, flow down and out of your body.

Let your awareness fall into the deep core of your torso, with the same feeling as letting yourself fall into the back and arms of a big, soft easy chair.

Taking slow full breaths, imagine that as each breath goes out, you sink deeper and deeper until you feel like you are merging with the earth. That's as grounded as you can be.

Phase 2: Closely Placing

Open your eyes halfway, so that your eyelids block the upper half of your field of vision. Focus your attention only on your posture and the sensation of your breathing, the feeling that your torso is filling with air as you breathe in, and then emptying as you breathe out.

When you realize that your mind has wandered into a series of thoughts, just think, "Back to here and now." Return to focus on your posture and breathing, without judging or criticizing yourself for becoming distracted.

Phase 3: Sensing

Open your eyes fully. Focus your attention on your vision, hearing, and bodily sensations, one after the other. Notice as much as you can, without mental commentary. You will discover that when one sense is in the foreground of your awareness, all the others move to the background.

Phase 4: Environmental Awareness

Leave your eyes fully open. As your breath moves out into the space in front of you, be open to the environment around you. Your mind can move to different objects of attention—sights, sounds, smells, sensations, and even thoughts—as long as they are in the here and now.

Again, when you realize that your mind has wandered into a series of thoughts, just think, "Back to here and now." Return to focus on your posture, breathing, and environment, without judging or criticizing yourself for becoming distracted.

Continue the practice of opening out and resting in spaciousness with each outbreath. In that way, you can experience thoughts and other sense perceptions clearly and distinctly as they arise.

Phase 5: Expansive Awareness

With eyes wide open, looking straight ahead, be aware of the environment around you. With each successive outbreath, expand the scope of your awareness. Imagine that your awareness opens out to the horizon, then to the sky, and then beyond the sky into outer space. Finally, imagine that your awareness extends in all directions, farther than the farthest star, and rest in that infinite openness for as long as you can.

Phase 6: Ending the Practice

Traditionally, each session of mindful awareness practice concludes with an aspiration. In your own words, affirm that you will be as mindfully aware as possible throughout the rest of the day or evening. You can also aspire that your practice will benefit both yourself and others.

"When you practice, fix your posture and align it so your body is a lightning rod between sky and earth. Then relax. Let your past dissolve into the earth, let your future dissolve into the sky, let the present moment dissolve with your breath—and then let go of everything you just did. Stare directly into space and relax your mind. Whatever happens, don't be concerned."

—Vajra Regent Ösel Tendzin,

Chariot of Liberation

Mindful Awareness in Action

A young man was traveling through the countryside. He stopped at the monastery of a Zen master with whom he had studied many years earlier. He was looking forward to having the master see how accomplished he had become in his practice, and that he was now himself a teacher.

It was monsoon season, and he wore rain shoes and carried an umbrella. He left them in the vestibule and entered the sitting room to meet the master. After exchanging greetings, the master asked, "Out in the vestibule, did you leave your umbrella on the right or left side of your rain shoes?"

Not being aware of how he had left his belongings, the new teacher realized he had more work to do in cultivating his practice of mindful awareness.

Mindful awareness in action means being completely present and attentive to whatever you are doing, and bringing your attention back to the task if your mind wanders. You can practice mindful awareness in many simple daily activities. Brushing your teeth, making your bed, getting dressed, setting the table, doing the dishes, sweeping the floor—any of these is a great opportunity to practice mindful awareness in action.

Eating, drinking, and exercising with mindful awareness will be the foundation for success in your weight-loss program and for your overall health and well-being.

By becoming more fully aware, you can recognize your patterns, enabling you to reinforce your successes and learn from your mistakes. Since mindful awareness is the ability to fully experience the present moment without self-conscious judgment, it provides an opportunity for discovering things about yourself that you may not have noticed before.

Mindfulness of your actions gives you more self-control. For example, you might open the fridge to get a bottle of sparkling water, see a leftover piece of pie and—before you know it—you've eaten it. Mindful awareness provides the time and space to reflect before you take action, decide whether or not it's worth the calories, and avoid the pain of regret.

Mindfulness of your speech and thinking is critical for combating the self-defeating rationalizations and justifications common to dieters:

- Once I start, I can't stop without finishing the whole bag.
- I can't help it, that's just the way I am.
- I'm tired, I'll exercise twice as much tomorrow.
- Yes, I had a donut. But it's not like I ate a half-dozen of them like last time.

With mindful awareness, you can hear yourself but choose *not* to believe what you're saying.

Practice Mindful Awareness in Eating:

Start with something simple, like a bowl of cereal or berries. Sit in good posture at the table, hands in your lap, the bowl of food in front of you. Moving very slowly, observe all of your movements in as much detail as you can, without comment or judgment. Slowly reach out and pick up your spoon. Scoop up a small spoonful of food. Bring it to your lips and put it in your mouth.

Set the empty spoon back onto the table and return your hands to your lap. Chew slowly, noticing flavor and texture, until you've finished that bite.

Repeat the process a few more times, increasing your speed until you're moving at as close to a normal pace as you can and still be mindful of your actions.

You may discover that you're moving very gracefully, doing everything in a very elegant way. This mindful awareness of movement is the same training that's used in the various Zen arts of Japan. My teacher, Chögyam Trungpa, described it as the expression of art in everyday life.

> *"When walking just walk,*
> *When eating, just eat."*
> —Zen Proverb

POINTS TO REMEMBER
FROM PART 2

- Time and Space to Respond, not React
- Be in the Here and Now
- Your Mind is More than Your Thoughts
- The Nature of Change
- The NINJA System™
  - Necessary Intention
  - Non-Judgmental Awareness
- Commitment to Your Intention
- Non-Judgmental Weigh-in
- Phases of Mindful Awareness Practice
- Mindful Awareness in Action

3

Taking Less In

Three Too's and Three S's

The *Three Too's* are obstacles to Taking Less In
- Eating **Too** Much
- Eating **Too** Fast
- Eating for **Too** Long

They are habits that prevent you from losing weight and keeping it off.

The *Three S's* make it easier for Taking Less In
- Smaller Portions
- Slower Eating
- Stop Eating Earlier

They are habits that support you in losing weight and keeping it off.

The Natural Order of Eating

The *Three Too*'s—eating *too* much, *too* fast, for *too* long—can be traced back to human survival instincts that were necessary in the distant past. Food was scarce. Our ancestors were hard-wired to eat as much as they could. As fast as they could. For as long as they could. When the food was gone, they stopped. Eating wasn't a matter of choice.

In modern society, when the danger of starving for most of Sus is gone, we get to choose how we relate to food. If we want to lose or maintain our weight, we need to be aware of our deep-seated eating impulses.

We need to recognize the Three Too's in our eating habits and apply the remedies of the *Three S*'s: eating smaller portions, eating more slowly, and stopping earlier. You can use the *The NINJA System* to change even deep-seated habits.

It's Not Your Hunger

For our ancestors, hunger carried with it the real possibility of starvation. Hunger pangs were more than an unpleasant feeling; they were a danger signal.

We are still hard-wired that way, with an innate negative response to the sensation of hunger. It triggers fear and anxiety. Being hungry is a bad feeling that we have to get rid of. We panic and want to eat—the sooner the better!

It feels natural when we're very hungry to say, "I'm starving!" Really? Unless you haven't eaten for days, and you won't be eating anytime soon, you're not starving.

Remember, it isn't even *your* hunger you are reacting to; it's the hunger of your great-great-great-great-great-great-great-grandparents.

Their instinctive, impulsive reactions to hunger—eating too much, too fast, for too long—are no longer necessary, and are in fact detrimental to your health and happiness. One step in overcoming the *Three Too*'s is changing your attitude toward hunger. When you feel a little bit hungry between meals, it's not something to be afraid of.

If you imagine that being a little hungry means you're out of fuel and starting to burn fat, it might not feel so bad. If you imagine that being a little hungry means your stomach is contracting, that might not feel so bad either.

Historically, losing weight was a danger sign while storing fat was good for survival. But your goals are the opposite. To support your weight-loss program, you'll want to choose to feel a little hungry rather than feeling stuffed. You'd rather lose weight, feeling lighter and thinner. You want that preference to override the instinct to consume calories that turn into fat.

It's possible that a change in attitude can even affect you on a cellular level. If you think of burning fat as a good thing, and that you don't need to conserve it as a resource, then the message you can imagine your metabolism gets is, "Burn, Baby-fat, Burn."

[*Important Note:* This attitude toward hunger is NOT for anyone with an aversion-type eating disorder. If you suffer from any eating disorder, it's important to consult a qualified medical professional.]

Are You Truly Hungry?

"You have thoughts, but you are not your thoughts. The practice is to recognize unhelpful thoughts and hear them—but not listen to them!"

—from the chapter "Know Your Mind"

Just because you have the thought, "I'm hungry," doesn't mean it's true.

Are you truly hungry? If you think you're hungry for a cookie, but wouldn't eat an apple instead—you may really *want* a cookie, but you're not really hungry.

Mom: *Johnny, eat your peas and carrots.*
Johnny: *I can't. I'm full.*
Mom: *Oh, I see. Then I guess you don't have room for ice cream.*
Johnny: *NO! I have room for dessert, just not for peas and carrots.*

There are different kinds of appetite that masquerade as hunger:

—Are your eyes hungry?

Does the picture of a deep-dish pizza on TV have you picking up the phone for a delivery? Do you really need to take everything that looks good at the buffet, or are your eyes too big for your stomach?

—Is your nose hungry?

Do you smell French fries as you're walking through the mall and head for the Food Court, even though you already had lunch? Do you smell popcorn and get in line, even though the movie has started and you just finished supper?

—Is your mind hungry?

Did you notice that it's past your usual lunchtime, think, "I'd better have something to eat," and make a beeline for the fridge? Even though you're no longer hungry, do you think, "I should finish what's on my plate."

Sights, smells, and thoughts about eating can trigger your appetite. They can make you think you're hungry, even when you're not.

Remember to use mindful awareness to take a step back and recognize what you're actually experiencing. That will give you the space and time to choose how to respond rather than react.

Before you eat, ask yourself, "Am I truly hungry?"

Try This:

Go through a checklist when you think about eating, and ask yourself, "Am I truly hungry, or:

- Are my eyes hungry? Does what I want to eat just look good? Would I feel the same about eating something healthier instead? Do I need to take that large a portion?"
- Is my nose hungry? Is the smell of food triggering a craving? Is it something I had planned to eat?"
- Is my mind hungry? Am I eating because of the time? Am I eating because others are eating? Am I eating for comfort from stress or emotions?"

Eating Like Cats and Dogs

Cats and dogs live on their instincts. When it comes to eating, cats have a regulator. Dogs don't.

Put a bowl of food in front of a cat. The cat takes a little sniff of the food, and if it's not hungry, it won't eat. If it is, it'll eat until it's no longer hungry. Cats eat to live.

Put a bowl of food in front of a dog. The dog will push past you, eat all the food in the bowl, finish the food that's still in the cat's bowl, and then beg for more. Dogs live to eat.

Dogs don't eat because they're hungry, they eat because they're eaters. They eat as much food as they can, as fast as they can, for as long as they can. They are hard-wired that way.

We need to remember that the instincts to eat too much, too fast, for too long are habitual reactions to our ancestors' hunger. Eating like dogs worked for them, but it doesn't work for us.

We need to eat smaller amounts, slower, and stop sooner. We need a new response to hunger. Eating like cats works better for us.

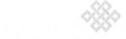

How Much Is Enough?

There's a big difference between feeling "no longer hungry" and being "totally full."

Americans say, "I'm stuffed," or "I couldn't eat another bite." On the other hand, the French use the expression, *je ne suis plus faim*, meaning, "I am no longer hungry." That is a much healthier way of determining how much is enough.

It's difficult to know how much food is enough when we are given enormous portions at restaurants, offered unlimited trips to the buffet, and tempted by supermodels in bikinis eating triple-bacon-cheese burgers bigger than their heads.

We stuff ourselves because of our habits of eating too much, too fast, for too long. It doesn't have to be that way. With mindful awareness, practice eating more slowly. This can include taking short breaks now and then. This helps you to recognize how full you're getting. Using *The NINJA System*, develop the habit of stopping when you're no longer hungry, instead of when you feel stuffed.

You can be fully satisfied without being completely full, and you will feel much better.

NINJA This:

Half an hour after each meal rate two things: 1) how full you think you are (0-100%), and 2) how your stomach feels (5=great; 0=terrible). Notice how you feel when you eat until you are really stuffed. Notice how you feel when you stop as soon as you are no longer hungry. You will start to prefer eating less because you would rather feel better after you're done. Eating less means you'll weigh less—and you know from the Weigh-Less exercise how good that feels.

Good to Know:

Your stomach doesn't actually shrink but you can feel like it has. If you're used to stretching your stomach by overeating, it will take longer before you start to feel full. The opposite is also true. If you get used to eating smaller amounts by stopping sooner, you'll start to feel full sooner, too.

Give It Time to Sink In

Think of the way the gas gauge registers as you fill the tank of your car. The pump clicks off at what seems to be three quarters.

By the time you drive away from the station, the gauge catches up, and you see that the tank is full.

Our bodies work the same way. It takes time for our minds to catch up with how full our stomachs are—up to 20 minutes! We need to give it time to sink in if we want to stop before we're stuffed.

Try This:

Split your normal helping of each dinner item into thirds. After you've eaten one third of each, take a break for a few minutes and reflect on how full you feel. If you're still hungry, eat another third, wait, and reflect again. You might discover that you need far less food to reach "no longer hungry" than you thought.

Helpful Hints:

- Take a break between courses, or after every few bites. You can relax with a few deep, mindful breaths. The more slowly you eat, the sooner you'll realize that you've had enough.
- Before dessert, take a 20-minute walk or some other break to give your brain the time to register how full you are. If you're no longer hungry, it will be easier to choose to skip dessert.

These tips are especially important for buffets and family style meals, where you're likely to both eat more, and eat more quickly, than you usually do.

Say No to Seconds

Taking less in means making a change in attitude. Instead of being concerned about not getting enough, you start to prefer not taking too much. You make the choice to "say no" when it comes to eating too much, too fast, for too long.

Several years ago I decided it was time to lose some weight because I got on the scale and the dial hit 200 pounds—and kept going. I decided to go on a diet but wondered, "What would happen if, instead of depriving myself of anything, I eat whatever I want, just not so much of it?"

The first step I took was making a commitment to "say no to seconds."

It wasn't that I always took seconds; rather, it was an expression of my intention to take less in. It was also a reminder of how stuffed I often felt when I went back for more. And if I ate slowly and mindfully, there was plenty of taste and texture satisfaction.

This proved to be an easy way to get over any inertia and resistance there was to dieting. It was a simple, gentle way to cut back on calories that didn't restrict my choices.

At the beginning, I took a good-sized portion of everything, to be sure I'd get enough. But, because my intention was to take less in, I started taking smaller and smaller portions. Soon I even chose to use a smaller plate.

It was moving me in the right direction, but I decided there was more I could do.

When a Snack Is Not a Snack

I made a commitment to also "say no" to unplanned snacking. And to remember that feeling a little hungry for a little while wasn't such a bad thing.

Instead of eating between meals, I'd have a glass of water. There are three benefits to this strategy:

- It's good to drink plenty of water to keep hydrated; after all, our bodies are more than half water.
- You might actually be more thirsty than hungry; thirst can masquerade as hunger. Drink water to take care of your thirst and your hunger will often disappear as well.
- Even if you are a little hungry, a glass of water will take the edge off by putting something in your stomach.

If the nutrition program that is best for you includes five or six smaller meals, or having something to eat between your three main meals, there's no problem. Just change your language. Don't call the snack a snack.

Instead, call it a *planned small meal*. Then you can "say no to seconds," "say no to snacks" (anything other than planned meals), and drink plenty of water.

Try This:

- To get a little extra entertainment from your glass of water, use a straw.
- For extra texture, drink sparkling water.
- For extra taste, drink naturally-flavored, no-calorie sparkling water.

Just Wait a Minute—or Five

Has this ever happened to you? You were hungry, prepared your lunch, and the phone rang. You took the call, got engaged in chatting and twenty minutes later you saw your sandwich still sitting there. Your hunger had taken a back seat to the conversation.

If you feel hungry and are thinking about having an unplanned snack, call a timeout. Give yourself a little space and time to respond rather than react. Reflect on your intention to "say no" to snacking. Remember that a little hunger is not something you have to be afraid of (or panic to get rid of).

Deciding to wait a little longer before you start eating will give you a sense of power over your hunger, a choice of how and when you respond to it.

Think, "I can wait five minutes," have a drink of water, and occupy yourself with a task that puts your hunger in the background. When your hunger returns, repeat this delaying tactic until it's time for your next planned meal. However, don't wait too long and get too hungry—you might react by overeating.

If you find yourself in this situation more than once, adjust your schedule or add a planned small meal in between your main meals.

Helpful Hints:

- The Job Jar: It's easier to stall your hunger if you're engaged in a task. Keep a "job jar" on the kitchen counter, and pick something to work on instead of eating.
- The Nap-Snack: When you start to feel hungry in the afternoon, check to see if you are actually beginning to feel tired or sleepy. If so, try taking a nap instead of a snack: a "nap-snack." Find a comfortable spot for a little 10- or 15-minute snooze. When you wake up, have a drink of water and carry on with your day.

You Have to Say No Sometime

"I can't have chocolate in the house. No matter where I hide it, I can hear it calling me. 'I'm over here. Come and eat me. Eat me now!' The only way I can shut it up is to eat it."

—A Dieter's Lament

Snack foods are usually loaded with salt, sugar, and/or fat, which makes us crave them. And that craving makes it hard to stop eating them once we start.

Ask yourself, "Am I truly hungry and willing to eat something healthy, or do I just have a craving for a candy or chips?" Remember that a craving for snack food is probably not real hunger.

If snack foods call to you when they are around, you'll find it easier to "say no" in the supermarket aisle and keep them out of the house.

Whether it's saying no to seconds at a meal, saying no to snacks, or saying no at the supermarket—at some point you just have to say no.

Practice This:

When you start dieting, do the Weigh-Less exercise at least once a week. It will remind you how good it is to feel lighter and strengthen your resolve to "say no" to unplanned snacking.

Erase and Replace:

If you don't want to "say no" to quantity, *erase* high calorie foods and *replace* them with lower calorie foods. For example, you can erase the side of fries and replace them with a side salad. Even with dressing on it, the salad has a lot less calories. *The NINJA System* can reinforce your positive choices. Give yourself a check mark each time you erase an unhealthy food choice and replace it with a healthy one.

You Are Not Your Cravings

One day, my teacher decided that it was time to take a break from sweets. He quit cold turkey. Just like that.

A few days later, he was sitting at dinner with a few of his students. It was time for dessert, and a lovely piece of his favorite chocolate cake was set in front of him. Then a piece was served to each guest. At that point I remembered that my teacher had quit eating sweets, so I said, "Excuse me, sir, would you rather we skip dessert, and have the cake taken away?"

He said, "No, it's okay."

Puzzled, I asked, "But doesn't it bother you to have it sitting there in front of you?"

He thought for a second, and then said, "No, not really," which puzzled me even more.

"But doesn't it make you want *to have some cake?"*

"Yes, but I don't take it personally."

Cravings are a kind of emotion. They are expressions of desire. You can work with your cravings the way you work with your thoughts in mindful awareness practice. Just because you crave something, doesn't mean you have to react to it.

When you are craving a particular kind of food, simply be aware of the feeling without acting on it. If you give it time, a craving will pass.

For example, after a meal you might feel like you really have to have something sweet. Then the doorbell rings and a package has arrived. You get the scissors and open it, finding the new sweater you had ordered. You head to the bedroom to try it on and your mind is no longer on food. What happened to the craving? It passed, just like every other wave of feeling or thought that appears on the ocean of your mind. If you don't take your cravings personally, you don't have to react or give in to them.

Practice This:

When you feel a craving for something, stop to look deeply into it.

Taking your mindful awareness posture, do a body scan to dissolve extra tension. Let your mind drop into an internal awareness of your feelings and let go of any mental storyline about them.

Ask yourself: "Where in my body do I feel the craving? How strong is it in each place in my body? Is it steady, is it vibrating, does it change into different sensations?"

Does the quality of the craving change if you tense up rather than relax? As you're observing it, is it getting stronger or is it fading? Is it connected to a flavor—sweet, sour, salty?

By making a craving the focus of your observation, you create some separation from it. When you don't identify with a craving, you're not compelled to react to it. You take away its power. You'll recognize that you *have* a craving, but you are not your craving.

Is It Worth the Calories?

It might be the bread in a basket, a side dish of potatoes, or a dessert on the menu. It could be a pastry at the coffee shop, or the baked goods in the break room at work. Whenever you have mixed feelings about whether or not to eat something, first ask, "Is it worth the calories?"

If the answer is yes, go ahead and enjoy it. If the answer is no, just say no.

To decide whether a food is "worth the calories," you need to know what you're dealing with. It's not hard to look up the numbers on your mobile device. Calorie counts are always printed on packaged foods, and more and more restaurants are making them available.

One morning in a coffee shop I was thinking about having a zucchini walnut muffin. It seemed to be a healthy lo-cal option, more like a salad than a sweet. But it was nearly 500 calories—even more than the chocolate fudge brownie! I asked myself, "Is that muffin worth the calories?" Knowing it would take more than two hours of brisk walking to burn those off, it was easy to say, "NO!"

Don't be swayed by addictive cravings for sugar, salt or fat. Taking a moment of mindful reflection will help you to let the craving subside and make a healthier choice.

Try This:

Water has zero calories. It's *always* worth it. Drink a glass of water before your meal. It will help you to take smaller portions and stop sooner.

Shrink the Window

The remedy of stopping sooner applies not only to *what* you're eating, but *when* you're eating as well.

Keep your eating to a limited range or window of time each day. Research shows that people who do so are less likely to gain weight, and more likely to lose it, when compared to people who eat at all hours.

Shrinking the window of when you eat is sometimes referred to as "intermittent fasting." You are fasting from the end of one day's eating until you start again the next day.

The ideal window of eating seems to be eight or nine hours, but there were still good results when eating remained within a 12-hour period. And it even worked when there were occasional slips in the schedule.

Try to stop eating less than twelve hours after you break your fast in the morning. For example, if you started breakfast at 7 a.m., do your best to plan your day so that you finish dinner by 7 p.m.

For those whose schedule means a late dinnner, if you don't finish eating until 9 p.m., try to wait before starting breakfast until 9 a.m. (Tea or coffee don't count, if you skip the milk or sugar.) When you can make the window of eating a little smaller, that's even better.

A common saying among doctors and nutritionists is, "If you want to lose weight, go to bed a little hungry." It makes sense— you don't burn up as much fuel while you're sleeping as you do during your daily activities.

However, going to bed so hungry that you can't sleep is counter-productive. So don't take this to an extreme. Your program might include one small planned meal in the evening. If you can, schedule it early enough to keep your eating in the twelve-hour window.

A "midnight snack" may be a long-standing tradition in your home, but it's time to turn the light off on this one.

NINJA This:

Write EATING LATE on your *Ninja* notepad, with the Necessary Intention of stopping earler. With Non-Judgmental Awareness, enter the time you stop eating each evening. You'll find yourself planning to finish earlier. Also, once you've made your entry for the evening, knowing you'll have to cross it out and enter a later time will help you resist going back for more to eat.

Helpful Hint:

Brush your teeth right after you're done with supper. It will make you think twice about having that evening snack, knowing you'll have to brush again.

Just Eat

*Two Zen students were telling each other about their teachers.
"My teacher is a great master who does amazing things. With
three strokes of his sword, he can cut an apple off a tree and slice it
into quarters before it hits the ground. He can shoot an arrow into
the center of a target, then split that arrow with a second one."*

*The other student said, "That's pretty good, but my teacher is
a really great master who does really amazing things."*

"What can he do?" asked the first.

*"When my teacher walks, he just walks. When he sleeps, he just
sleeps. When he eats, he just eats."*

Mindful eating encompasses an entire way of approaching food
that will help you take less in. It prevents the *Three Too's* and
supports the *Three S's*. You'll eat more slowly and stop sooner.
You'll eat smaller amounts but enjoy what you're eating more.

It seems pretty simple—when you eat, just eat. The problem
is that we hardly ever just eat.

In this day and age, multi-tasking is the norm. It's rare that
we are only doing one thing at a time. Television, emails, and
social networking—we feel like we have to keep up with all
of them while we're working, playing, and eating. Otherwise
we're wasting time. So while we're eating we're also watching

television, checking emails, or surfing the web. We try to save time by eating while walking between classes or as we're driving to work (dangerous—don't do it!).

However, multi-tasking isn't really possible. The mind can only focus on one thing at a time. Everything else goes to the background. If your mind is elsewhere while you eat, you aren't paying attention to the flavor of the food or to how full you are. Before you know it the food is gone, but you hardly tasted it. You ate too fast and too much. You feel stuffed, but not satisfied.

There's a problem on another level. A connection develops between eating and what you've been doing while eating. Before long, when you start to watch television or surf the web, you'll also feel the urge to get something to eat. And mindless eating in front of a screen of any kind will undermine your intention to take less in.

Instead, when you eat, just eat. Take the time to eat more slowly, with mindfulness of the taste, temperature, and texture of each bite. You'll make better choices about what to eat, get more satisfaction from it, and recognize when you no longer feel hungry.

Helpful Hint:

Pre-set your table with placemats, dishes and silverware. Keep it an uncluttered, device-free zone. Make it a "mindful awareness zone," where you can slow down and fully appreciate the joy of eating as meditation.

Set Them Down

Here's a surprisingly powerful technique to encourage mindful awareness during meals: To slow yourself down, set your utensils down.

Often, as soon as we've put a spoonful of food in our mouth, we start loading up the next bite. Instead, after taking each bite, gently set your utensils down and chew until that bite's finished.

I hardly tasted anything because I was always busy loading up my fork or spoon, staying one bite ahead of myself. Setting my utensils down helped me enjoy everything I was eating, one bite at a time.

If you are clenching your fork, you may also be clenching your jaw. When there is tension in your jaw, you can feel it in your shoulders, neck, and forehead. It even extends to your arms, chest, back and the rest of your body—a tense jaw can make your toes curl!

You may find that when you are holding on to your utensils, you are also holding your breath! When you relax your grip, your whole body relaxes and it's easier to breathe.

I noticed that when I set down my knife and fork, I relaxed and leaned back in my chair between bites. And without thinking about it, I was chewing more slowly.

NINJA This:

To develop the habit of SETTING THEM DOWN, have your notepad with you at the table. Each time you realize you are holding on to your utensils and starting to take some food for the next mouthful while you're still chewing, put the utensils down and make a tally mark. You'll soon be more aware and more consistent at setting them down with each bite.

Mind Your Peas and Chews

Eating mindfully means enjoying the texture and savoring the flavor as you first taste the food, as well as while you're chewing. Chew slowly and thoroughly, swallowing little by little, until that bite is gone.

There are many practices and traditions that encourage chewing each bite anywhere from 15 to 40 times.

There are several benefits of this practice:

- You get more flavor from each bite, so you can be satisfied with smaller portions.
- You eat more slowly, so you recognize when you are no longer hungry and can stop sooner.
- You are processing the food more thoroughly before it reaches your stomach, so you can digest it better.

Be the Last to Finish

If you find that you are often the first one finished with your meal, you can practice mindful eating by trying to be the last person at the table with food on their plate.

Not only will you get all the benefits of eating more slowly, you may find that you enjoy the social aspect of a meal in a new way.

When you are talking, just talk. When you are listening, just listen. When you are eating, just eat.

Savor the Flavor

The better your food tastes, the more fulfilling the experience of eating will be. Just a few bites of something really delicious can be more enjoyable than a plateful of less flavorful food. High quality foods can be expensive, but they are worth it if you can eat smaller portions of them and be even more satisfied.

You also get more satisfaction from food that looks beautiful. That's why arrangement on the plate is such a big deal in fancy restaurants.

It will help you take less in if you opt for quality foods, and take a few extra moments to prepare and set them out in an attractive way.

With mindful awareness, focus on the taste and texture of each bite. Eating more slowly helps you savor the flavor, which makes it easier to be satisfied with smaller portions.

Helpful Hints:

- Take smaller bites. You get to enjoy the flavor longer when you take two or three small bites rather than one big mouthful.
- Take it slow. Remember to put your utensils down after each bite. Slowing the momentum of eating gives you the time to relax and fully appreciate the flavors.
- Stop sooner. When you savor the flavor, just a few bites of a treat can satisfy you. Save what's left to enjoy another time.

Try This:

See how many bites you can get from a 100-calorie portion of one of your favorites—two, three, four, or even more. That's a great way tĺo get maximimum enjoyment from a special treat with minimum damage and minimum guilt.

Eat What You Really Want

"Pooh always liked a little something at 11 o'clock in the morning, and when Rabbit said, 'Honey or condensed milk with your bread?' he was so excited that he said, 'Both,' and then, so as not to seem greedy, he added, 'But don't bother about the bread, please.'"

—A.A. Milne, *Winnie the Pooh*

You know what you like, so choose to eat less of what you don't like.

For example, Leslie enjoys a pasta dinner, but the sauce is the best part. Taking a smaller portion of noodles and using a little more sauce reduces the calories by one-third or more.

Pat likes the texture and flavor of bread and mayonnaise in a sandwich, but what's in the middle is less important. A low-cal option is to substitute a stack of lettuce and a slice of tomato for the calorie-rich meats or cheeses.

Making your sandwich topless—even PB&J—is a good tactic if you don't care about the bread. Cutting out a slice of bread will save you some calories.

Identifying what you really want to eat is an opportunity to introduce mindful awareness into your meal planning process. It's a strategy that pays off twice: you get more satisfaction while you take less in.

Try This:

Think of five of your favorite dishes and decide what you really want from each. Be creative in coming up with lower calorie versions. Use more of the ingredients you like best and eliminate or reduce the rest.

If you find success with these new and improved recipes, go ahead and create satisfying lo-cal versions of all your regular dishes at home. When eating out, it can't hurt to ask for substitutions that get you more of what you really want.

It's Not Food

I've always really liked the smell and taste of bacon, but it gives me indigestion. I had to make a choice: both or neither. Were several hours of discomfort worth a few seconds of enjoyment? No, thank you!

Rather than telling myself that I wasn't allowed to eat this tasty food, it was easier for me to move it into a different category. Bacon was no longer food to me. I convinced myself that it was the same as chewing on aluminum foil—not a pleasant sensation.

Processed food has lots of preservatives and other chemicals. When I see those on the label, I regard them as plastic rather than food. And I'd rather not eat plastic.

Whatever food you want to avoid, it will be easier if you regard it as metal, plastic, or some other inedible substance. Just tell yourself, "It's not food."

Rule of Thumb

Your stomach's ordinary capacity is about one quart. If you eat more than that, the capacity will expand to accommodate the greater volume (up to three or four times as much). If you get used to stretching the limit, you'll need to eat that much more before feeling you're no longer hungry. You'll get in the habit of eating too much, and gain weight. To lose weight, you need to do the opposite. Stick to smaller portions and you won't overload your stomach.

Here are a few fun rules to help you choose the right portion sizes for:

- Veggies—be a two-fisted salad eater
- Fruits—one fistful is fine
- Protein—as big as your open palm
- Carbs—cup them in one hand
- Chocolate—no larger than your thumb
- Dessert—wave goodbye with your empty hand!

Try This:

Using measuring cups or spoons, portion out foods you commonly eat and put them on a plate. Now you can see what each amount looks like. Practice until you can recognize your ideal portion sizes without using the measuring tools.

Optical Illusions

To support your intention to take less in by taking smaller portions, use smaller plates. Whatever portions you serve your-self will look bigger on a salad plate than on a dinner plate.

Using a smaller plate at the brunch buffet kept me from taking
too much when my eyes were bigger than my stomach.

It's good to use smaller utensils as well. You'll take smaller bites using a teaspoon instead of a tablespoon. That's a recipe for mindful eating, better digestion, and taking less in.

Contrasting colors also make portions look bigger. You can serve brown rice on a white plate, and white rice on a brown plate. It's an optical illusion, but even knowing that, it still feels like you're getting more blueberries when they're served in a yellow bowl.

Pre-Pack to Prepare

Pre-packing is an important strategy for portion control. This works especially well for any foods that you can freeze. For example, break a pound of lean hamburger meat into four quarter-pound patties and freeze all but the one you'll be eating for dinner that night.

Some things are easier to portion out after cooking. A cooked sweet potato can be cut into thirds. Wrap the two extra pieces separately and freeze them for future meals.

Taking the time to separate portions before you eat makes it easier to resist the temptation of going back for more. You have time to reflect on the choice you're making. And that gives you an opportunity to respond based on your commitment to the *Three S*'s, instead of giving in to the *Three Too*'s.

Helpful Hint:

When dining out, ask for a take-away box *before* you start eating. Pre-pack all but your ideal portion size—you'll feel better, stay slimmer, and have plenty left for another delicious meal tomorrow.

Put It Away

After you have your morning toast you won't think twice about popping in a second slice if the loaf, butter and strawberry jam are still sitting there on the counter.

Once you have taken a serving, put the rest of the food away before you start eating. Don't leave the pot on the stove, the casserole in the oven, or the pizza box on the counter.

Have a container ready to pre-pack whatever you won't be eating. Put it away and you won't be as tempted to have seconds.

Putting it away sets up an extra threshold you have to cross to keep eating—it gives you the time and space for awareness and discipline to help you stick with your program.

Eat Outside the Box

Okay, so there was a commercial break in the show I was watching, and I felt like having something sweet. I hit the pause button and headed for the kitchen. Poking around in the fridge and the freezer, I saw the ice cream. I took off the top, but said to myself, "Three bites, I'm only going to have three bites."

I started around the edges, where it was a little softer. I thought, "That wasn't really three full bites — more like one and a half. I can have three more of those."

I saw that after scooping around the edge, there was a bump in the middle. I forgot that I was counting bites and leveled it out.

The edge where I was holding the carton had melted, and I knew it would get icy when I put it back in the freezer, so I thought, "I'm just going to clean it up a little bit." But then there was a little bump in the middle again, so I evened that out.

Now I was on autopilot, eating from the middle, then the edge, middle, edge, middle, edge, until my spoon hit the bottom.

At that point I thought, "This isn't really worth putting back. Oh, what the heck, I'll just finish it off."

Have you ever been there? Done that? It could be a pint of ice cream, a bag of chips, or a package of cookies. Whatever the container, it's easy to keep eating once we've started. We're especially susceptible if we're eating while we're watching television or surfing the web, mindlessly chomping along with the action. And we'll continue digging in until we reach the bottom. It's as if we're hypnotized from the repetitive motion and taste, and we'd dig all the way through the earth to the other side if it were made of ice cream.

Of course it's easier to eat out of the container. Why dirty a dish just to have a few handfuls of nuts? And there are only a few more chips in the bag, so why bother putting them in a bowl?

If you're coming up with an excuse for eating out of the container, remind yourself that just because you think it's a good idea, that doesn't mean you have to believe it.

Instead, make part of your Necessary Intention to eat outside the box—take what you want to eat out of the container, put it in a bowl or on a plate, and put the container away. Then enjoy your small planned meal!

NINJA *This:*

Write STOP EATING OUT OF THE CONTAINER on your *Ninja* notepad. Anytime you notice yourself eating that way, stop and make a tally mark. Soon that habit, and the pounds, will disappear.

The Clean Plate Club

A lot of eating happens after you're no longer hungry, but before you're full. Be mindful as you eat, and stop when you've had enough. Whatever's left can either be put away or thrown away. Don't feel like you have to eat every last bite.

It's an interesting choice point when there's just a little bit left. You're no longer hungry, but you're caught in the momentum of eating. If there's not enough to put away, you'll be tempted to finish it off.

Finishing off what's left is a common habit. Many of us have a natural aversion to waste. We may have been brought up with our parents telling us to be in the Clean Plate Club. It's hard to leave that last bite.

When my children were young, I gained weight because I ate all the food they didn't finish. I felt a little like a human garbage can, but couldn't get myself to waste food by throwing it away. What was I thinking?!

Rather than feeling that you are wasting food, regard not cleaning your plate as a symbol of your ability to be able to stop when you want to. Resign from the Clean Plate Club!

Stopping before the food is completely gone doesn't mean depriving yourself. It's your positive choice if you are no longer hungry and would prefer not feeling stuffed.

In a restaurant, the server will often say, "Are you still enjoying your dish?" Use that question to ask yourself if you really are still enjoying it. "Do I need to eat every single bite now? Or am I no longer hungry?" Choose to take a doggie bag home, and you'll feel less discomfort and guilt after dining out.

Watch Out for These:

- Rationalizing:

    You might think, *"There's so little left, it's not worth putting away. I'll just finish it off."*

    Or, *"I don't know when I'll get back to this restaurant again. I want every bite I can get."*

    Remember that you don't have to believe it just because you think it!

- Momentum eating:

    Beware of the tendency to just keep eating because it's there, not because you need to, or even want to, eat more.

- Eating on the run:

    Catch yourself before grabbing "a little something" as you walk by the fridge or cabinet on your way out the door. That's an unplanned snack of extra calories.

- Nibbling:

    Beware of tasting as you cook. Three nibbles add up to a bite, three bites add up to a portion, three portions add up to an unplanned meal. And that adds pounds.

I couldn't figure out why I wasn't losing weight on my diet. Then I realized what it was. While baking a batch of cookies each week for my daughter's school program, I was mindlessly eating chocolate chips—one for the cookie dough, one for me; two for the cookie dough, two for me... Oops!

Split the Entrée

Yogi Berra, the quotable baseball star, was asked by a waitress whether he'd like his pizza cut into four slices or eight. He replied, "Better make it four — I don't think I can eat eight slices."

—Diet Humor

Restaurants are notorious for giving over-sized portions. Half of a normal entrée is often large enough for a full meal. So when you go out to eat, split the entrée. Share it with your companion. Or save a portion to take home with you. In addition to eating less at that meal, your lunch is already packed for tomorrow!

Appetizers are often more interesting than entrées, and smaller. So why not make one of those your meal? If there's an entrée you'd like, ask if you can order the appetizer size.

My husband and I went out Saturday morning to one of our favorite brunch places. We ordered two different dishes, ate slowly and each enjoyed half our meals. We then packed up what was left and took the packages home. Sunday morning we warmed up the leftovers, and enjoyed each other's dish from the day before. We each got two great brunches for the price (and calories) of one!

POINTS TO REMEMBER
FROM PART 3

- Obstacles: The Three **Too**'s
  - Eating **Too** Much, **Too** Fast, for **Too** Long
- Remedies: The Three **S**'s
  - **S**maller Portions, Eat **S**lower, **S**top Earlier
- Don't be afraid of feeling a little hungry
- Recognize if you are truly hungry
- Stop when you are no longer hungry rather than totally stuffed
- Give your brain the time it needs to catch up to your stomach
- Say No:
  - To Seconds
  - To Snacks
  - At the Store
- You are not your cravings
- Decide if it's worth the calories
- Shrink your window for eating
- Slow and mindful eating
- Set your utensils down
- Know your ideal portion size
- Prevent over-eating with:
  - Smaller, colorful dinnerware
  - Pre-pack, put away, and portion out
  - Split the entrée or order smaller

PART 4

Challenges to Taking Less In

Watch Your S.T.E.P.

Stress

Temptation

Emotion

Personality issues

These present challenges to your positive choice to take less in and lose weight. You truly have to watch your *STEP* and be vigilant in supporting your intention to "Say No" with the tools of Mindful Awareness, Maitri, and *The NINJA System™*.

The Challenge of Stress

Stress creates a general sense of anxiety. We lose touch with our body; we're tightly wrapped up in the thoughts racing around in our head—totally "uptight." Everything seems to be moving faster. So we move faster to catch up, but can't, like a dog chasing its own tail.

Human beings are hard-wired to reduce anxiety as quickly as possible. For many of us, when faced with stressful situations that won't readily resolve, the fastest, easiest, and surest way to reduce anxiety is to eat it away.

If food calls to you in stressful times, you probably have the mistaken idea that eating will solve your problems. We've been conditioned to eat to soothe ourselves. My grandmother's solution for any upset was, "Eat something; you'll feel better."

Comfort food does make you feel better, and while you're eating you don't have to deal with what's stressing you out. Unfortunately, the relief is temporary.

Eating doesn't address the source of your stress, and you have to face it again when you're done. On top of that you've actually made it worse from the guilt of smothering your anxiety under a burrito. Not to mention the indigestion.

When you feel like an unplanned snack, ask yourself, "Am I really hungry, or am I just trying to escape the stress?"

Knowing that it won't solve your problems, but will add unhappiness the next time you step on a scale, is it really worth it to temporarily relieve stress with food?

Practice This:

The grounding practice of mindful awareness (see Appendix) is a direct antidote to stress. Deep breathing moves your energy down in your body. It slows the speed of your thoughts and helps you relax—"grounded" is the opposite of "uptight." When you feel stressed, and especially when you feel the urge to "stress-eat," take a time-out and do a few minutes of grounding practice.

NINJA This:

Erase your habit of stress-eating, and replace it with a healthy response.

Mark down an S each time you realize you are reactively stress-eating. Mark down an H each time you feel the urge to stress-eat, but respond in a healthier way, such as:

- A few minutes of the grounding practice;
- Taking a walk or other exercise;
- Starting on a bite-sized piece of a project that's been stressing you out.

When a Reward Isn't a Reward

Do you use food as a reward after you've completed a stressful job? Does the idea of food soothe you and calm out-of-control feelings?

Studies have shown that sugar cuts the stress hormone cortisol, so sugary comfort food actually can make you feel better. Temporarily.

If you're on a weight-loss program, rewarding yourself with something sweet often backfires. The sugar crash brings you down, and remorse for the binge brings up feelings of guilt and shame. These feelings can provoke further eating, and a disheartening cycle ensues.

If you're not careful, using food to reward yourself can end up being just the opposite: cruel, unintended self-punishment.

However, it's great to give yourself a reward that supports your weight-loss intention, such as adding to your wardrobe when you succeed in being slimmer and trimmer!

Altered States

Alcohol is an inhibition disabler and addiction activator that makes you say, "I want what I want when I want it." It makes you forget the past and not worry about the future, but not in a healthy way.

The soothing experience of having a drink makes you want another, and the inhibition suppressor in it makes you say, "Why not?" To paraphrase the great comedian Richard Pryor's comment on addiction: A couple of drinks can make you feel like a new man. The problem is: then the new man wants one.

Alcoholic drinks contain a lot of calories. Also, the cocktail snacks usually served with them are especially salty and fatty, making you want to drink more. Once you get on the drinking and snacking merry-go-round, it's awfully difficult to get off, so it's better to stay off.

In some states, recreational marijuana is legal, and presents an additional challenge. It reduces inhibitions and increases your appetite. It's not a coincidence that the feeling it gives you is called "the munchies!"

Both alcohol and marijuana make positive, healthy choices extremely difficult. There's a reason "intoxicated" contains the word "toxic."

When your inhibitions are suppressed, you may realize that you are overeating, but you just don't care. If you do indulge, do your best to have awareness of your "don't-care-ness."

With Friends Like These

It's hard to stay on your weight-loss program around others who don't share the same intention.

C'mon, one time won't kill you. Just one cookie won't hurt.
I'm going to have a snack, but I don't want to eat alone.

You're often going against the grain of social pressures when you make positive diet choices. This applies to being with a friend who doesn't understand how hard it is to lose weight, or with your mother who asks, "No seconds? What do you think I'm trying to do, poison you?" When everyone is having a second glass of wine or heading back to the buffet, it's hard to say, "No, thank you."

It can be embarrassing to ask friends and family not to offer you seconds or snacks. It takes discipline to resist social pressure.

Practice This:

Establish your intention before entering into group dining or drinking situations. Write down how much you plan to eat or drink, and if things get tough and you feel tempted to eat more than you planned, excuse yourself and take a little walk to gather your resolve. When you come back you'll be in a better frame of mind, and better able to resist temptation.

The Temptations

"The Temptations" aren't just a great Motown R&B group from the '60s. The temptations that lead you astray from your intention to take less in and lose weight are particularly challenging when:

- You're at a restaurant and the waiter just put a basket of yummy, warm, fresh-baked bread on the table as you are hungrily waiting for your meal;
- You're at a party with drinks being served and snack foods set out on every table;
- You're at work and there's a candy jar on the reception desk and free snacks in the break room. It seems like every week someone has a birthday celebration with cake and ice cream. And, oh, the parade of holiday baked goods that marches through the office.

What's a dieter to do?

It's important to be mindful and make positive choices. Take preventive measures by planning ahead.

Don't arrive too hungry at a restaurant, dinner party, or family barbeque. Drink a glass of water as soon as you arrive.

Be sure there are alternative, healthier foods available for you to choose. Call ahead—if they aren't being offered, ask if it's alright to bring your own.

NINJA *This:*

Before you go out, write down your plan for what you will and won't eat. Check off what you do eat and what you "say no" to.

Practice The Push-Aways

- At a party, when there are chips on the coffee table near you, push them away.
- At a restaurant, push the breadbasket away. If you are dining with fellow dieters, ask if they'd mind having it taken away (or not brought over in the first place).
- At work, when you can't push temptations away, push yourself away. Don't linger in the break room or anywhere that food is set out.
- At any meal when you've eaten enough to be no longer hungry, push away from the table.

Higher Calories? Higher Shelf!

What if you have kids and can't "say no" at the store?

If you have to keep some high-calorie foods in the house, put them on the highest shelf. There's no need for a cookie jar on the counter to tempt you.

Out of sight, out of mind. And beyond that, if you do remember they are there, it will take you some time and effort to get them.

That delay will allow you to be aware of the craving and not react to the impulse for an unplanned high-calorie snack.

For dessert I like a square or two of a chocolate bar. But I keep it on the highest shelf in the kitchen. That way I have to pull out the stepstool to retrieve it. So if I give in to the urge, at least I get some exercise!

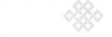

Beware the Buffet

If you are at a buffet, you're going to need to be mindful that seconds, or even thirds, are not only encouraged, but actually expected of you. If you're at an all-you-can-eat restaurant, you might feel as if you're not getting your money's worth if you don't keep going back as many times as you can.

A buffet is like the official headquarters of the *Three Too's*— the easiest place on earth to eat too much, too fast, for too long.

Here's how to apply the *Three S's* as a remedy:

First, make the Necessary Intention to take no more than two small plates of food.

Walk through the line without a plate to decide what you really want to try. That includes the dessert table—the most dangerous of all. Decide if any of the desserts are really going to be worth the calories. If so, plan on taking the smallest portion you can be satisfied with.

Next, on a salad-size plate, take just a bit of each dish that looked good enough to eat.

Eat your small portions slowly and mindfully. After you've tasted each one, and finished the ones you really liked, take a break for a few minutes. You may decide you've had enough, and can stop eating.

If you are truly still hungry, take your small plate back for another small portion of your favorites.

You'll have the satisfaction of enjoying the food you wanted while keeping to your weight-loss program. And feel very proud that you conquered the *Three Too's* in a very challenging setting.

Drive By the Drive-Thru

"What a revoltin' development this is!"
—from the radio and television series, *The Life of Riley*

The drive-thru window is one of the most unfortunate things to happen in the history of eating.

Not only does it inspire mindless, speedy overeating, but it discourages even the tiniest bit of exercise.

We zoom into the driveway, shout the order at the clown's mouth, pay our money, and grab our food. We take off with a fistful of greasy fries in one hand and a milkshake in the other, steering with our knees.

Eating while driving is bad for your diet and dangerous for everybody else on the road. And it can get you a ticket for driving while distracted.

So remember to drive by the drive-thru.

The BLAST Zone

It's tough enough getting through a normal, no problem day, particularly if you've just started a new diet or when you've hit a plateau. But your resolve can be in real danger when you enter the **BLAST** Zone:

Bored

Lonely

Angry

Sad

Tired

When you experience these emotions, you are especially vulnerable; your defenses are down and you aren't thinking clearly. It's hard to remember your intention to take less in.

One reaction to emotional intensity is to suppress it, and one way to do that is to eat. It's more than a metaphor that as you swallow the food, you swallow the emotion; as the food goes down and fills you, you are pushing the emotion down and burying it.

To protect yourself from getting **BLAST**-ed off your diet, employ mindful awareness and *The NINJA System*, as well as these helpful tactics:

The Three Practices

To work with emotions, it's necessary to have a perspective on your experience. If you are totally caught up in the emotion, you are completely reactive, with no space or time to make a mindful response. The following practices allow you to take a step back, regain your composure, make healthy decisions, and take positive actions:

1. Meditate: Take a few minutes to practice the stages of mindful awareness. It will calm the emotional intensity by pacifying the mind and settling the body.

2. Contemplate: Insight can't happen in the midst of emotional upheaval. Feel the texture of the feeling beneath the thoughts that accompany the emotion. When you drop the "story line" that supports it, the intensity fades and you have the space to think things through. Contemplate the circumstances that trigger emotional reactions and establish the Necessary Intention to respond in a healthier way.

3. Activate: With mindful awareness, put remedies that have worked for you in the past into action, or try the following suggestions:

Protection from the BLAST Zone

Bored: Don't use food for entertainment. Pick something from your to-do list. Clean out a purse, briefcase, or closet, catch up on some household chores or some reading, do a favor for an elderly neighbor. Check things off your to-do list and save calories at the same time!

Lonely: Don't use food to keep yourself company. Phone a friend, go for a walk (it's helpful to encounter nature, especially tame animals), or take an exercise class. There are also online forums and other resources that connect you with dieters facing the same challenges. (For example, Weight Watchers® offers its members a real-time online chat.)

Angry: Don't use food to stuff your anger down. Meditate, breathe, and ground yourself to be calmer and clearer. Don't suppress or indulge in your anger. Don't act it out or deny it. You can choose to burn it off, channeling the energy into creative, positive actions. Even better, write about your feelings. But be careful not to hit the send button!

Sad: Don't use food to cheer yourself up. Listen to uplifting music. Water your plants. Play with your pet. Depression usually makes you feel lethargic, so "move your mood." Decide to do one minute of exercise to get yourself going; the positive feeling can build momentum for a full session.

Tired: Exhaustion heightens emotionality and diminishes your ability to resist impulses, so food triggers are more likely to kick in. Studies show that when people get one-third less sleep than usual, they eat 600 more calories the next day!

Take a time-out and get some rest. Try meditation, yoga, or deep breathing. Do some light exercise; a little movement can get your flow going.

For all of the **BLAST** Zone emotions, feel them fully and relate with them using the Three Practices, rather than stuffing them down and covering them up with food.

NINJA This:

List the triggers that set off the **BLAST** Zones, and the remedies that work best for each. Notice, with Non-Judgmental Awareness, whether you react with emotional eating or choose positive, healthy responses. In that way you can change your habits to protect your weight-loss program when you find yourself in the **BLAST** Zone.

Helpful Hints:

- Imagine that a friend is struggling with a similar trigger and emotional reaction. If you were their coach, and they were eating to suppress that emotion, what would you tell them to do instead? Take your own advice, and put it into action.
- Arrange with a friend to be weight-loss coaching partners. When either of you get caught in the **BLAST** Zone, call each other for support.

Momentum Eating

Momentum has a quality of urgency. As in, "urge" for more. And more. Until you've eaten too much, too fast, for too long.

Our ancestors faced scarcity of food and weren't able to preserve leftovers. They almost always kept eating until the food was gone. So we have an innate tendency to do the same.

Salt, sweet, and fat are addictive triggers that can start and sustain the momentum of long, unfortunate binges. A potato chip company ad used to brag about that: "Betcha can't eat just one!" As the addictive taste fades, you have the urge to experience it again and think, "Just one more." And then more. And more. Until they're gone.

You're momentum-eating when you're mindlessly caught up in the rhythm of the repetitive movements, bite after bite after bite. That's why it's so important to set your utensils down between bites, and not eat out of the container.

Distractions make it even easier to get swept along. That's how you find you've eaten an entire tub of salty, buttered popcorn at the movies before you know it. Studies show that people eat even more watching action movies because of the excitement.

You're also momentum-eating when you start to feel full, but you still have eye hunger and smell hunger. And that last bite tasted so good. Especially if you're holding the food in your hand, like a burger or piece of pizza, it's hard to stop.

Try These Remedies:

- Put it away. Far away. Or give it away. Or throw it away. Or don't buy it in the first place. To stop addictive momentum, you have to "say no" sometime.

- Apply mindful awareness to recognize and catch yourself in mindless MOMENTUM EATING and *NINJA* that habit.

- Take a break. Pracitce stopping halfway through your meal for 60 seconds. That may lead to a longer break. A gap in the momentum of wanting more allows you to recognize that you may not need more. Remind yourself of your preference to feel lighter and slimmer, and save the rest of your meal for later.

Never Enough

"When you really need nourishment for your spirit,
filling your stomach isn't the answer."
—from the chapter "Be Kind to Yourself"

The Zen tradition has metaphors for different personalities. One of them, "Hungry Spirits," are beings that never feel full because their stomachs are the size of a mountain but their mouths are as small as the eye of a needle. This metaphor represents any state of mind in which one feels hollow and unfulfilled.

Any amount of nourishment is never enough. In fact, getting partial comfort only intensifies the frustration.

Eating to fill an emotional hole creates extra suffering because we are looking in the wrong direction for a solution. The problem is that our stomach is not what we need to fill. If the emptiness is in our psyche or spirit, we need psychological or spiritual nourishment, not more food.

I felt like I didn't matter to anyone, that I wasn't important in any way. I didn't know how to feel worthwhile by myself, so I tried to fill the hole in my soul with food.

I used eating to blot out the despair. It gave me something to look forward to, and some pleasure at the start. But as I continued to gain weight, eating also made me feel awful about myself. This cycle eventually became so painful that I couldn't live like that anymore. I sought out a therapist, and that was the start of healing.

To nourish your spirit, it's essential to have a non-judgmental attitude of maitri. Self-acceptance is the antidote to feelings of inadequacy and hopelessness.

"Your overweight self doesn't stand before you craving food. She's craving love."

—Marianne Williamson

NINJA This:

- You can erase the mental habit of giving yourself negative messages, even ones you have internalized from childhood or abusive situations. Write down the words that you most often use to describe yourself, such as UNWORTHY or UNIMPORTANT. Non-judgmentally make a tally mark each time you realize that you are caught up in those thoughts or feelings.

- To erase the habit of eating to fill an emotional hole, write down words like HUNGRY SPIRIT EATING and non-judgmentally make a tally mark when you catch yourself. Replace eating with meditation, yoga, or some kind of exercise.

Compulsive Eating

"I don't stop eating when I'm full.
The meal's not over when I'm full.
The meal's over when I hate myself."
—Louis C.K., comedian and compulsive eater

Some people look for opportunities to reinforce their negative self-image, so they eat themselves sick.

I went to a holiday party and couldn't leave the "cookie" room. I ate and ate until I was stuffed, then left with a doggie bag of cookies and ate those before reaching home. I had trouble sleeping because I felt shaky from the sugar, sick to my stomach, and equally sick of my compulsive behavior.

Do you feel powerless to stop eating? It may be that you want to eat until you feel bad about yourself. It's a painful way to confirm your feelings of low self-esteem.

Feeling bad about yourself keeps you in a negative kind of comfort zone. And when comfort foods are your primary stress or emotional coping mechanism—cookies, bagels, potato chips, ice cream—you can get stuck in an unhealthy cycle where your real feelings are never addressed. The problem is actually more about mentally beating yourself up than overeating.

There's a connection between self-sabotage and identity. When you do well, you feel it's lucky and just a matter of time before you blow it. When you slip, it's agonizing proof that you're just no good. The remedy for this is to shift emotion to the positive—a slip doesn't define you. Instead, take positive pride in what you accomplish, like putting things away before you eat, putting your utensils down while you chew, and turning down dessert because you'll feel lighter and better without it.

If you can shift your identity from negative habits to basic goodness, you'll be able to start breaking the self-defeating cycle of stress and overeating. Use mindful awareness and maitri to recognize and accept what you're feeling and where it's coming from.

You might feel like there is so much clay you can't imagine there could be any gold underneath. When there are deep issues that underlie an eating disorder, psychological and/or spiritual work may be necessary.

If your experiences are truly overwhelming, get the help you need to turn things around and uncover your gold.

Nature or Habit?

A Zen master was listening to a student complain about his uncontrollable temper. The student said, "I'm a very angry person. Please help me to change."

"Sounds like a big problem. Let's see this terrible anger of yours," the master demanded of the student.

"I can't show it to you. I'm not angry right now."

"Then when can you demonstrate it for me?" the master asked.

"I don't know. It takes me by surprise."

"This anger must not be your true nature. If it were, your anger would be available for display any time. If it's not there all the time, and you can't even summon it when you want to, obviously you are not an angry person."

To say that someone has a habit of compulsive eating doesn't imply that it's part of their nature. Calling them a compulsive eater does. Thinking about your own or others' behaviors in terms of habit rather than nature makes life much more workable.

This can be particularly useful in working with feelings of helplessness in relation to eating. When you find yourself deep in a half-gallon of ice cream, it's easy to feel like there's something deeply wrong with you. But if you recognize that you have a habit of compulsively eating ice cream—that is a behavior you can change. There is hope.

POINTS TO REMEMBER

FROM PART 4

- Watch your STEP:
  Stress, Temptation, Emotion, and Personality issues
- Don't use food as a reward
- Alcohol or marijuana suppress inhibitions and
  invite overeating
- To resist peer pressure and temptations,
  have a plan and stick to it
- Use remedies to protect yourself from
  the BLAST Zone:
  - Bored
  - Lonely
  - Angry
  - Sad
  - Tired
- Catch yourself to stop momentum eating
- Recognize that compulsive eating is a habit,
  not your nature
- If you're overwhelmed, get the help you need

PART 5

Burning More Up

"A bear, however hard he tries,

Grows tubby without exercise."

—Winnie T. Pooh

The Natural Order of Exercise

Just as there is a natural order to eating, so there is a natural order to human exercise that began long ago. Before refrigerators, supermarkets, and drive-thru windows, there was a constant struggle just to find enough food to remain alive.

And there was always output before there could be input.

Whether it was hunting, gathering, or farming, people always had to work before they could eat.

Life in earlier times simply burned more calories.

Now, however, we have to make a special effort to expend energy. When we don't, those unused calories are converted into fat, and we are converted into couch potatoes.

The technological strides we've made have caused the equation between taking in and burning up to become unbalanced. We need to find a way to bring back some of that natural order.

Balance the Equation

The old Zen master always worked alongside his students. Together they trimmed shrubs, pruned trees, and swept the grounds.

When he was eighty years old, his students worried that the physical labor was too much for him, but he denied their requests that he stop working. So one day, they hid his tools.

At dinner, he sat without eating. He just said, "No work, no food."

The next day he wouldn't eat at all. At each meal he said, "No work, no food."

On the third day, the students had no choice but to give back his tools. The master worked in the garden again and silently resumed eating.

We will never surrender our modern conveniences, so we must find a way to restore the balance between what we take in and what we burn up. To do this successfully, we need to make exercising a positive choice rather than a punishment.

The word "exercise" is not pretty or sexy, and it doesn't naturally fit into the box we label "pleasurable experiences." However, regular exercise has been proven to reduce stress, ward off general anxiety and feelings of depression, boost self-esteem, and even improve sleep. Exercise also strengthens your heart, lowers blood pressure, reduces body fat, and makes you look fit and healthy. Focusing on one or more of these valuable benefits, we make exercise something that we *want* to do.

Understand how much work it takes for your body to burn off calories. Schedule enough exercise to offset what you're eating. Or cut back on calories to match what you're burning.

Changing the equation is the only way to reduce your weight. Balancing the equation is the only way to maintain it once you've reached your goal.

Helpful Hint:

Chart the calories contained in the foods you like to eat and the calories you burn in the exercising you like to do. *NINJA* any habits you need to change in order to balance the eating/exercise equation.

How Long Is Enough?

Exercise will help you lose weight, and it will also help you keep the weight off. However, your schedule limits how many calories you can realistically expect to burn off in a day, week, or month.

A person who weighs 140 pounds would need to walk briskly for two hours to burn off 450 calories. Can you fit a two-hour walk into your schedule on every day that you eat a 450-calorie snack? In this case, "skipping" is one of the best exercises you can do, if it's extra calories that you're skipping.

While the bulk of any weight loss will be attributed to taking less in, this should not undermine your resolve to either strengthen or adopt an exercise routine. The benefits of exercise are important for keeping weight off once you have established your dieting program and begun to lose some, if not all, of the pounds you have targeted.

Keep an exercise log in tandem with your eating log. This will allow you to see the progress you're making, and apply *The NINJA System* to optimize your exercise routine.

NINJA *This:*

Set your daily schedule for exercise. At the end of each day, record how many minutes you exercised compared to your planned amount. It will encourage you to follow through on your plan more regularly, or show you that your plan needs to be adjusted.

Exercise Mindfully

Before each session, do a little deep breathing and relaxation with a body scan, to prepare you for stretching and warming up.

While you're exercising, mindful awareness helps you coordinate your breathing with your actions. That will make your exercise session more efficient. Using the exercise you're doing as the object of your mindfulness in action can improve your mental focus and stamina.

Be mindful of how tired you are getting, and any strains or pains you're feeling, to keep from exceeding your limits and hurting yourself.

Record the length of your session and the exercises you did. Let your success be your reward and inspiration for the next session.

NINJA This:

When beginning an exercise program, you are bound to feel some resistance. By applying mindful awareness to your experience, you can recognize the inertia holding you back from a new and challenging project. With that recognition, you can use *The NINJA System* to set the Necessary Intention to exercise a certain amount, and use your Non-Judgmental Awareness to record your progress. Use a pedometer, fitness tracker app, or any other device that helps you in your journey.

Good to Know:

Be aware of the tendency to use a completed exercise session as a rationalization for indulging in a high-calorie binge. Remember the balance—it won't help your weight-loss program if you burn up 500 calories exercising and then wolf down a 600-calorie ice cream sundae.

Overcoming Procrastination

A common obstacle to exercising is procrastination. "I'll do it later" always seems to sound better than "I'll do it now." Anticipating the discomfort of an exercise session is reason enough for us to find an excuse to avoid it. If we're feeling comfortable we will not go out of our way to feel uncomfortable.

It's also difficult to imagine the future benefits of exercising when all we are faced with is the immediate unpleasantness of huffing and puffing, sweating and swearing.

However, we can create situations where exercising seems as if it just happens naturally, by making it quick, easy, regular, and even fun.

Make It Quick

When it's time for a session, if you feel resistance, try to give yourself a good reason why you can't exercise for just five minutes. If you have a good reason, relate to it. If you can't come up with one, get started right away.

This keeps you from making excuses—not enough time, too tired, don't like to sweat, and so on. You could waste five minutes arguing with yourself about whether to exercise or not. Instead, try the following routine:

- Find five minutes in your daily schedule.
- Put it on your calendar.
- Do your exercise.
- Do the same thing every day.

When you're ready, you can add more short exercise sessions each day, or increase the length of your session.

This allows you to overcome resistance, begin exercising in a gentle way, and eventually build a full-length exercise routine.

Make It Easy

The easiest exercises are ones you can do without planning or special equipment. *Casual exercise* means adding an element of exertion to the way you do everyday activities. There are lots of ways to be more active throughout the day.

One place to start is to walk as much as possible. Walk up the stairs instead of taking the elevator. If you live or work in a high-rise, at least walk up the first three flights. Park your car at the other end of the lot or down the street.

One of my favorites is "The Stand Up." Whenever you sit down, stand up again—one, two or even three times—before you remain seated. If this reminds you of the Weigh-Less exercise, get your bag of groceries and do it!

More Examples of Casual Exercise

- While waiting for the elevator, an appointment, a bus, or a train, do wall push-ups or gentle squats.
- Walk around the house and do simple chores on tip toes.
- If you're watching television, lift some light weights, do isometrics, or ride a stationary bicycle.

Make It Regular

By exercising at times that fit your personality and your schedule, you greatly increase the chance that you won't be skipping your walks, jogs, or spinning sessions. "Morning people" like to just get up and go; "late risers" not so much. When selecting a daily time to exercise, take into account all of the excuses that you might rely on to avoid it, and pick the time that is the easiest to commit to and continue with.

Helpful Hint:

Schedule walks at times that you struggle with cravings. Give yourself a little "earn it before you eat it" inspiration by exercising before a meal.

Make It Fun

Most people complain about exercise because they see it as a burden, hardship, or unwanted intrusion into an otherwise pleasant day. Framing it as something you'd rather not do makes it easy to find a way not to do it. On the other hand, choosing activities that you enjoy makes it easier to include exercise in your weight-loss program.

You may like to walk or swim, to ride a bike or dance. Whatever kind of movement it is that makes you feel good, do it. If you find that you get bored doing the same routine day after day, change it up. Whatever you do, you'll do more of it if you make it fun.

Just Get Your Gear On

Here's a way to get you through the inertia and over the resistance you may have to exercising.

Tell yourself, "I'm not going to exercise. I'm just going to get my gear on." This way, you're not anticipating the negative feelings that you associate with exercise. It's not much strain to get your gear on.

Change your clothes. Put on whatever you wear for an exercise session, and take out whatever gadgets you use—straps, weights, balls, or rollers. Just putting your sweats and sneakers on is a step in the right direction, even if it's a baby step.

Now you've got your gear on. Tell yourself, "It would be a waste of time to put my gear on and then just take it off again. I'll stretch and warm-up." After that, tell yourself, "It would be a waste of time to get my gear on, stretch and warm-up, and then just quit. I'll exercise for three minutes."

When you're almost done with the three minutes, tell yourself, "I'll just do two minutes more to make it five. Then I can count it in my exercise log." By the time you've done five minutes you will have worked through the initial resistance. You may even start to feel the endorphin effect (the brain chemical that gives you a good feeling from physical exertion). Before you know it you'll have done a half-hour or more. And that's how just getting your gear on helps you do a full exercise session.

Helpful Hint:

Have exercise clothes that are comfortable and colorful, that fit well and are fun to wear, so that you'll really want to get your gear on.

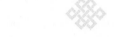

Phone a Friend

Don't go it alone! Many people find that once they begin exercising with a partner, they skip sessions far less frequently. It's great to have a friend that you know will be there to not only accompany you, but to encourage you, and be encouraged themselves. Knowing that your partner's waiting for you will help you get over the resistance to exercising on those days when you just don't feel like it.

Don't Hurt Yourself

Once there was a lion cub that wished he were as big and strong as his father. But he didn't want to wait until he grew up. So he tried to imitate his father in every way he could. The father lion walked with big slow steps, so the cub walked in what he thought were the same big slow steps. His father roared a great roar, so the cub made the sound that he thought was a great roar. Then his father jumped across to the other side of a deep ravine.

When the cub tried to imitate him he tumbled down and down until he plopped into the bushes at the bottom, a bit bruised in both body and pride.

An obstacle to burning more up is the pain of exercise. Already overburdened joints and long-unused muscles call out, "Stop exercising, you'll hurt yourself!" As if you needed another reason to put off something that you have a hard time getting into.

Take a gradual approach. Trying to do too much too soon will result in hurting yourself and could set your program back by days, weeks, or even months.

Start with low impact ways of burning calories. For example, a stationary bike will put less stress on knees and ankles than will running. Isometrics may be less stressful than free weights.

Accept where you are, and begin from there. Trying too hard to progress too fast will only get you hurt.

Second Wind

Many people feel tired shortly after they start an exercise session. They decide, "I don't have the energy today," and stop before they really get going.

It's a common experience during running, cycling, or other activities that require sustained effort over a period of time, to feel that you're just about out of energy at a certain point. But if you continue on a bit longer, suddenly you have a second wind, a feeling of renewed energy that encourages you to keep going.

The way to bring this about is to scale back the intensity of your actions a little bit and continue on at that reduced level. Soon you'll shift into another gear, feel like you have more energy, and be able to complete your exercise session for the day.

Enjoy Your Endorphins

Being able to enjoy exercise is extremely valuable for success in your weight-loss journey. The terms "endorphin rush" and "runner's high" sound appealing, and it's possible that you have experienced one or both of them.

Endorphins are also known for being released in response to eating certain foods like chocolate or macaroni-and-cheese.

You may know these kinds of endorphins all too well, but all you really need to do is replace them with exercise endorphins.

When I ride my bike for half an hour, I'm left with a general sense of well-being. I guess that's what they mean by endorphins. Looking forward to that experience encourages me to want to get on the bike again and again.

POINTS TO REMEMBER
FROM PART 5

- Understand how much you need to exercise to burn off a given amount of calories
- Do the Weigh-Less exercise to remind you of your intention
- Exercise mindfully
- To overcome resistance, start with short sessions
- Gradually build up to a full-length exercise session
- Take the opportunity to do casual exercise whenever possible
- Schedule exercise for the time of day that works best for you
- Make exercise a regular a part of your life

PART
6

Keeping on Track
In Dieting and In Life

"At any moment you have a choice
that either leads you closer to your spirit
or farther away from it."

—Thich Nhat Hanh,
Venerable Zen Master

How Does a Mouse Eat an Elephant?

Long ago in Japan, a student came to a master of Kendo, the art of the sword, and said, "If I become your devoted student, how long will it take for me to master the sword?"

The master replied, "Perhaps ten years."

"That's a long time," said the student. "If I try really hard, how long would it take me?"

The master replied, "Oh, maybe twenty years."

The student was shocked. "First you said ten, now you say twenty years. What if I try as hard as I can?"

"Well," said the master, "in that case it will take you thirty years. Someone as impatient for results as you are will probably take a long time to accomplish anything."

Ambition is a powerful motivator. It is a key element of progress toward any goal. But it is a double-edged sword. It can be dangerous if not channeled and directed properly. With ambition comes urgency, which often creates tunnel vision. Being overly focused on results can make you blind to pitfalls on the path to progress. In your urgency for improvement, you might fail to notice the messages your body is sending you. If you don't recognize your body's limitations, you can push yourself too hard and get hurt.

Drastic diets usually don't work. When extreme dieters try to lose too much weight too quickly, it results in either health problems or a rebound reaction of abandoning the diet altogether. Because these diets don't change a person's fundamental relationship to eating, the weight goes back on because old habits come right back.

Question: "How does a mouse eat an elephant?"
Answer: "One bite at a time."

If your goal is to lose 30 pounds, approach it little by little. Begin with a five-pound target. If you're starting at 160—don't think about 130, just focus on 155. Once you reach that, 150 becomes your new goal, and 155 your ceiling. With each successive five-pound stage, give yourself a little longer to reach your objective.

Halfway to your goal, start using two-pound targets and ceilings. Know that there are ups and downs along the journey. Work within your goal and ceiling range. When you are in the lower half you know you're doing well; if you drift back into the higher half or past your ceiling, it's time to take a look at what's going on.

Don't be so hard on yourself when you see your weight fluctuate higher. Beating yourself up won't help you stick with the program. Just notice, non-judgmentally, what has changed in your eating or exercise habits. Refocus your efforts to stay on track.

In this way, slowly and steadily, you'll reach your target of weighing 30 pounds less.

Goldilocks

Most of us are familiar with the fairy tale of "Goldilocks and the Three Bears." When she entered the bears' house, Goldilocks encountered three versions of everything: two extremes and one in the middle. The Papa Bear's chair was too hard, the Mama Bear's chair was too soft, but the Baby Bear's chair was just right. The Papa Bear's soup was too hot, the Mama Bear's soup was too cold, but the Baby Bear's soup was just right.

When beginning a new diet, your daily life may get complicated, making it easy for you to respond by going overboard. You either attack the day with the attitude of "I have to do everything perfectly" or you resign yourself to "forget this, I've got no chance." Neither of these will prove fruitful, and the new diet program will go out the window faster than you could have imagined.

Likewise, after you've had some success with your program, don't get ahead of yourself and relax your discipline. If you've hit a plateau, don't start overdoing it and get yourself sick.

Zen is often referred to as The Middle Way, being free from the two extremes—neither a life of pure self-indulgence nor one of continuous self-denial. The Buddha taught the middle way to a musician who asked, "How should I hold my mind in meditation?"

"Just the way you would tune the strings of your instrument. Not too tight, not too loose, just so."

It can be very hard to pinpoint what is "just so," but it's not hard to say when something is too far in one direction or another. We can use freedom from the extremes to find the middle way.

Not Too Excited, Not Too Depressed

A student went to his teacher and said, "I don't know what to do. I am terrible at mindful awareness practice. I'm preoccupied with the past half the time, the future the other half. I can't just be present and relax. I'm very frustrated, and getting nowhere."

Without seeming the least bit concerned, the teacher said, "These things come and go. Keep practicing."

After a month, the student requested another interview. "You were so right. Now my mindful awareness practice is excellent. I feel settled and calm, aware and present. I'm very confident, and really getting somewhere."

Without seeming the least bit impressed, the teacher said, "These things come and go. Keep practicing."

The #1 New Year's resolution is to lose weight and get fit. That shows how many people recognize the need for starting a weight-loss program.

Unfortunately, it is also the #1 most commonly broken New Year's resolution. Of those who do lose weight, only a small percentage keep the weight off for the long run.

To remain effective over a lifetime, with all its ups and downs, a weight-loss program can't just be a quick fix. It must provide you with tools that will support you in continuing the new direction of your life. It must become a part of your life, so that it can't be sabotaged by a bad day or one wild and crazy weekend. Do your best to not get too excited about dropping a pound, and not too depressed if you slip and put on a pound.

Beware the places and times that send you into the **BLAST** Zone and back to old habits. Relying on mindful awareness and *The NINJA System* will help you maintain the good new habits you've developed.

Especially when you reach a goal, either in one of your stages or your ultimate target, there's a danger in getting complacent and feeling like you've finished. The next phase of your journey, maintaining your weight, has just begun.

Diminishing Returns

When you first begin a new diet, it may seem that you are moving along at a good pace. Later, there will be times when you feel like you're doing everything right, but you see no change when you step on the scale. It's easy to feel disappointed, but you have to remember that you've been doing something really good for yourself.

You've worked really hard and stayed focused on your Necessary Intention, but hit the dieting wall or plateau. Stick with your program. Don't give up or give in to old habits. Engage your new habits, like the Weigh-Less exercise, with greater frequency.

If the calories you burn equal the calories you eat, you will maintain your weight. To lose more weight, you need to either decrease the calories you eat or increase your physical activity.

Understand that weight may not be the only measure to consider. You know your program is working because your clothes fit better or they're roomier, and people have been commenting on how good you look. You can also look at pictures of yourself when you were a lot heavier, and appreciate what you're accomplished so far.

You're changing your relationship to food and eating, and this is for keeps. It's a lifestyle change that will reap many benefits.

So, when the pace of progress slows down, don't lose heart.

Now, Where Was That Scale?

Sometimes when things go well we get complacent. We either forget to log our meals, neglect our afternoon walk, or simply don't get on the scale.

If we're struggling with our discipline, we can get discouraged or frustrated. We are embarrassed to log what we're eating, don't feel like going for a walk, and are afraid to get on the scale.

Without a way to right the ship, we just might give it up completely.

Set up a weigh-in schedule that works for you. If you do a lot of your dieting during the week and are a little more relaxed in your eating habits on the weekends, you may only want to weigh yourself every Friday.

If part of your plan is to weigh yourself every day, don't listen to the thoughts that are trying to talk you out of it. It's a slippery slope when you skip a day. You say, "I'll do better, and weigh myself tomorrow." But then you don't do as well as you thought you would, so you skip another day. And pretty soon your program is falling apart.

Helpful Hints:

- The best intermediate target for you is one that is inspiring rather than discouraging.
- Accept that your weight is not going to steadily decrease; you'll have your ups and downs.
- Do the Weigh-Less exercise as a motivator and reminder of your intention.

Keeping It Off

"How did I let this happen again?!"

—from an interview with Oprah Winfrey

When we reach our target, why is it then so hard to maintain our ideal weight? Rather than a new healthy lifestyle, we usually approach a diet as "something we go on." Therefore, it will eventually be "something we go off."

If we haven't used the *Positive Choice Model*, dieting feels like being forced to give up things that we like. So a reservoir of desire grows, a longing to have those experiences again. We can't wait to go back to not feeling deprived. That's why most people find it harder to keep the weight off than to lose it in the first place.

The first phase of your program is completed when you reach your target weight. The next phase is maintaining that weight and sustaining good health and fitness. That's your program for the rest of your life. A lag in discipline and motivation can lead to regaining the pounds you've worked so hard to lose. It is surprisingly easy to slip into old habits, and before you know it you're asking, "How did I let this happen again?"

We need vigilance to maintain our intention, and continually work with the habits that arise from our deep-seated reactivity to hunger, stress, temptations, and emotional triggers.

It can't be a one-shot deal, a short excursion into dieting. Maintaining your ideal weight is a lifelong journey, an ongoing healthy relationship with eating and exercise.

The Yo-Yo Way of Life

Examine your eating patterns. Do you lose weight, then put it on again, then lose it again, going up and down like a yo-yo? Some people alternate drastic diets and binges. Others lose weight gradually, then slowly put it all back on. It doesn't matter whether it's fast or slow—you're in a self-perpetuating cycle.

It's time to ask yourself some questions:

If it's so painful, why do I keep doing it? What am I getting out of behaving this way? If this is what I've become, do I want to remain this kind of person?

"Hitting bottom" is a phrase common to twelve-step programs. It's the point at which someone decides that they can take it no more. For some, this may be what has to happen for them to develop the motivation to not only lose weight, but to keep it off.

I felt I had hit bottom when I realized that my eating behavior was affecting every aspect of my life.

Regarding your weight loss program as a prison term can turn you into a dieting yo-yo. You lose weight on the diet, but when you've done your time you go back to the old habits that made you overweight in the first place.

Repeatedly losing weight and regaining it again can not only be demoralizing, but can be bad for your heart. Studies have shown that repeated weight fluctuations are associated with seriously increased risks in relation to heart disease.

To step out of that cycle, you need to step into a new and healthier way of life.

Helpful Hint:

If you've gone on a binge:

- Write down everything you ate, as painful as that may be.
- Use it as motivation to strengthen your discipline.
- Journal the triggers, feelings, and circumstances that gave rise to it.

With Non-Judgmental Awareness, note the rationalizations, environments, and emotions that lead to and enable your binges.

More Curious Than Afraid

This is a true story, told by my dear friend Pema Chödrön in her book, *Start Where You Are: A Guide to Compassionate Living*. It happened in southern California in the early 1900's.

A Native American man, the only surviving member of his tribe, had been hiding on an offshore island for many years. He was discovered and brought to an anthropologist at a nearby college who took him into his care. His name was Ishi, and the anthropologist taught him English and various things about the modern world.

One day the anthropologist wanted to take Ishi to San Francisco. They went with some friends to the station to get the train. As it neared the platform, Ishi slipped quietly behind a column. The others were boarding the train and noticed him peeking around the column. They motioned to him to come along. He slowly came out and climbed aboard.

Later the anthropologist asked him how he enjoyed the train ride. Ishi told him that his tribe thought trains were iron monsters that roamed the countryside and ate people.

The anthropologist expressed his surprise that even though he thought the train was a monster, Ishi got on board with little more prompting than a wave from his friends. "How did you have the courage to do that?!" he asked.

"Well," said Ishi, "Since I was little I was taught to always be more curious than afraid."

Often, as we approach a new level of success, fear appears. For some it's the fear of failure; for others it's the fear of success.

The fear of failure creates anxiety. To escape from that anxiety we might sabotage ourselves and go off our diet at the slightest discouragement. We succeed in avoiding the anxiety of not reaching our goals, but we never allow ourselves a chance at true success.

Fear of success comes from imagining what will be expected of us and not believing that we will be able to live up to those new standards. Again, we find ways to undermine our efforts with self-sabotage to avoid the anxiety we anticipate.

We can't deny our fears, we can learn to go beyond them. If we accept our fears rather than run away from them, we have the opportunity to respond rather than react to them. That is true fearlessness.

Like Ishi, we can take an attitude of openness and curiosity about our lives no matter what we might find in the future. This allows us a path through our fears, and provides us with a real chance for lasting success.

As the saying goes, "Life is like a turtle. If you don't stick your neck out, you never get anywhere."

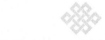

Cover the Roads with Leather

In ancient India, there was a queen whose feet were very sensitive. She complained constantly about the kingdom's roads, which were rough and rocky. Finally, the queen decided she would have all the roads covered with leather, so that wherever she wanted to walk, her feet would be comfortable.

She invited the best contractors to bid on this formidable project. One replied, "I can do the job, but it will cost all that is in the kingdom's treasury." Another said, "I can cover the roads with leather for half of what is in the treasury."

Then the queen's old chambermaid whispered to her, "I can do the job for 10 rupees. I'll just strap a piece of leather under each of your feet, and you'll be walking on leather wherever you go."

There are several reasons we complain. First, we'd like something done about a situation. More often than not, it's beyond our control. For example, we might be unhappy that even a small order of fries has so many calories, but complaining won't change things.

We also complain to protect our egos. We feel better if we can blame something else. We want an excuse; it's not our fault if we ate too much.

But complaining only makes a bad situation worse. Adapt yourself and your state of mind to whatever you encounter. Accept the conditions and make the best of them. You often can't control what happens to you, but you can always control how you respond to it.

Whether it's the free donuts in the break room at work or a family reunion at an all-you-can-eat buffet, respond to the situation in a positive way, without complaining.

My teacher, Ösel Tendzin, gave his students this simple but powerful instruction:

Don't complain.

About anything.

Not even to yourself.

Everybody Makes Mistakes

It's hard to be kind to ourselves after making a mistake, despite the fact that we know everybody makes them. I use the following exercise in my corporate workshops to illustrate this point. I ask everyone to imagine that a good friend has slipped on his or her diet program, like going to a party and eating a lot of food they'd usually stay away from. Then I ask them to insert their friend's name as they say the sentence, "That's okay, [insert friend's name], everybody makes mistakes."

I tell them to imagine they are saying it in an actual situation, being as encouraging and enthusiastic as they possibly can. When asked how that felt, people say it felt good to be able to give support and comfort to a friend.

I have them repeat the same sentence, but this time imagining that they went on the binge themselves, and inserting their own name instead of their friend's. When they say the sentence in this way, most of their voices are barely audible. Many people have painful looks on their faces. Some laugh nervously to avoid the tension. Some say they feel their chests constrict or their throats tighten up.

Most of us find it much easier to be kind to a friend than to ourselves. It's easier to tell a friend, "That's okay, everybody makes mistakes," than to say it to ourselves. In general, people give themselves a really hard time, and have a really hard time giving themselves a break.

If you're struggling with your diet, try not to add insult to injury with negative self-talk. Recognize and accept what happened, and resolve to do better next time. Treat yourself like you'd treat your best friend, with positive comments of encouragement. Be kind to yourself.

Let Go of the Past

Once there were two monks walking along a path through the woods. When they came to a stream, they encountered a young woman, dressed in fine silks, unable to get across without ruining her clothes. One of the monks offered to carry her on his back. She climbed on, they all crossed the stream, and on the other side he set her down. She thanked him, and the two monks continued on their way.

The monastery to which these monks belonged had a rule that they were not allowed to touch women. The other monk was horrified that his brother in the order had broken this rule, and was agonizing about it as they walked. He thought, "How could he violate his vows like this? Will he confess? Should I tell the abbot? Will they throw him out? Will I get in trouble, too? Why did he put me in this situation?" And he got more and more upset.

Finally, after they'd gone about a mile, he stopped abruptly and shouted, "How could you do that?!"

"Do what?" asked the first monk.

"How could you touch that woman?!"

"Oh, her? I set her down when we got across the stream. Why, my brother, are you still carrying her?"

Like the monk in this story, when we get upset by something, we can carry it with us for a long time. It's as if we can change the past by replaying it in our mind and conjuring up a different result.

Being caught up in the past makes it impossible to do your best in the present. With mindful awareness, accept the circumstances and let go of guilt and self-hatred as soon as you can.

This applies both to eating more, and exercising less, than you had planned.

My teacher, Ösel Tendzin, offered this four-part remedy for dealing with regret:

1. Acknowledge what happened and take responsibility.
2. Learn from it and do what you can to repair any damage.
3. Work on changing your habits to prevent it from happening again.
4. Let it go and don't waste another moment on it.

Sandwich of the Day

You can take the principles in this book and apply them to more than dieting. You can apply them to life.

Think of each day as a mindful awareness sandwich. The two pieces of bread are how you start and end each day.

You start the day with intention and end the day with recollection. Your activity is the filling, somewhat different every day, sandwiched in between intention and recollection.

First thing in the morning, before you do anything else, take three deep breaths to clear your mind and rouse your energy. Mentally establish your basic intentions for the day. Plan to be as mindfully aware of your thoughts, speech, and actions as possible.

Commit to your diet program and the *Three S's*: smaller portions, slower eating, stopping sooner.

You can also include the intention to maintain positive self-talk and good communication with others. That's one slice of bread.

Throughout the day, be as present as you can, coming back when you wander into daydreams of the past or future.

At the end of your day reflect on how you did. That's the other slice of bread. To what extent did you fulfill the Necessary Intentions that began your day? It's not a contest; you didn't win or lose. Just recollect what happened with Non-Judgmental Awareness.

To the extent you were not mindful, think that you'll do your best to be more tuned in. If you slipped a little, recognize what triggered it, what you could have done better, and reaffirm your intention. Had a major "oops?" Don't punish yourself, just plan to take a fresh start tomorrow.

Whenever and wherever you did well, take satisfaction in that. However much you maintained your mindful awareness, be happy that you and others benefited from it.

Having completed the sandwich of the day, sleep well.

PART 6
POINTS TO REMEMBER

- No drastic diets. Slow and steady.
- Take the middle way.
- Don't get too excited, or too depressed.
- If you hit a plateau, don't lose heart.
- Keeping the weight off is often harder than losing it. Make your weight-loss program a way of life, not a temporary diet.
- Cultivate a fearless attitude, don't complain, let go of the past, and be kind to yourself.
- Start and finish each day with a positive attitude.

The principles presented in this book provide a tried and true path that will benefit you in all aspects of your life. Taking them to heart will allow you to fulfill your potential and realize your goals.

It is my hope that what you have read has allowed you to tap into your unconditional confidence and reveal the gold that is your true nature, and that it will help to make your weight-loss journey and whatever you experience in life ever more rewarding for you and your companions.

APPENDIX

This is the expanded version of the phases of a practice session presented in the chapter "Practicing Mindful Awareness."

Although the instructions following are sufficient for beginning the practice of mindful awareness, if one wishes to delve deeper, it is important to have personal instruction from a qualified teacher.

Also please note: Persons with respiratory issues should consult a heath professional before doing any breathing exercise.

Phases of Mindful Awareness Practice

The practice of mindful awareness trains you to:

* Pay better attention to what you are doing.
* Maintain that attention for longer periods of time.
* Notice more quickly when your attention wanders.
* Return more sharply to the here and now.

The *mindful* aspect of the practice is being precisely focused on what your body and mind are doing in the here and now, whether you are sitting still or performing an activity. The *awareness* aspect of the practice is being tuned in to the environment in which your thoughts and perceptions come and go, moment by moment.

Combining the precision of mindfulness and the perspective of awareness, you can return to the present when you wander, and be fully responsive to whatever arises in your experience.

Take Your Seat

Find a place where you can sit uninterrupted for as long as you intend to practice. For a beginner, it is helpful to find a quiet place, and practice for short periods of time. Until you strengthen your concentration, any hustle and bustle around you will be distracting. When your focus is stronger, you will be able to maintain your mindful awareness while in the midst of a busy workplace, during an intense conversation, or with a group of friends at a restaurant.

While this practice is traditionally done sitting cross-legged on a cushion, most people find it easier to sit on a chair or footstool. If you use a chair, sit in the center of the seat without leaning against the back. It's helpful to have your knees level with or lower than your hips, to prevent strain on your legs and back. Your feet can be flat on the floor, or loosely crossed in front of you.

Hold Your Posture

Practicing mindful awareness is best begun in sitting position because when we stand there is a tendency to move, and when we lie down there is a tendency to fall asleep. People sit up straight when they're paying attention. That's why we say "we're on the edge of our seats" when we are very interested in something. Simply taking this position with good posture promotes mindful awareness.

Good posture makes it easier to stay attentive, and easier to breathe. You'll want your spine to be upright but not rigid. The back of your head can gently extend up, so that your chin tucks in slightly. To get the proper feeling of this, stand with your shoulder blades and hips against a wall, and gently bring the back of your head to the wall.

Let your sternum (breastbone) move very slightly up and forward, while the middle of your back moves very slightly backward and wider. This expansion of your torso takes pressure off your lungs, allowing you to breathe more easily and fully.

Sitting up straight but not stiff is ideal, so feel as if your spine is a tent pole and the rest of your body is like canvas hanging loosely from the top of the pole.

Let your arms hang straight down from your shoulders, and place your hands palm down on top of your thighs, just behind your knees. Let your jaw muscles soften, leaving your lips lightly closed.

Grounding

Having established proper posture, the next step in mind training is the process of getting grounded in three stages:

First, gently close your eyes. Let any excess tension, beyond what you need to hold your posture, flow out of your body by mentally scanning from head to toe. With the intention to soften areas of tension, just touching them with your awareness will start to dissolve them, like sunlight melting snowflakes in the morning.

Notice any tightness in your:

- face, jaw, and neck,
- shoulders, arms, and hands,

- chest and shoulder blades,
- belly and lower back,
- hips, thighs, calves, and feet.

Let the tension you encounter dissolve as much as it will, and feel that it flows down and out of you, into the earth.

Second, let your mind move down into your core. Most of us feel that our mind is somewhere in the front of our head, because much of what we use to engage our world—our eyes, ears, nose and mouth—are positioned there. With your eyes still gently closed, let your mind fall backward, toward the back of your skull, with the same feeling as letting yourself fall into the back and arms of a big, soft easy chair. From there, let your mind drop slowly down through your body. Feel that you are settling downward along the front of your spine, like a leaf slowly drifting down to the bottom of a pond, past your throat, heart, and stomach, to your deep core just below your navel.

The third phase of grounding is merging with the earth through deep, rhythmic breathing. Imagine that as each breath goes out, you sink deeper into the seat you're on. As you inhale, just stabilize that feeling. Sink deeper and deeper each time you exhale, eventually feeling like you are merging with the earth—that's as grounded as you can be. Your breathing will become slower and softer as you become more settled and relaxed.

Close Placement of the Mind

When you train a dog or horse, you first need to tame it. To do so you give it a very short leash, holding it close to you so you can pull it back quickly when it starts to stray. You need to tame your mind in the same way; therefore this phase of practice is called "close placement." By focusing your attention only on your posture and your breath, you keep your mind placed close to you, on a short leash.

It is traditional to use the breath as the basis for training in mindful awareness. Our breath is somewhat under our control (for only so long), but also happens when we're not thinking about it. It is part of the environment coming into us, and part of us going out into the environment.

In this phase of practice you focus your attention on your body as you breathe in and out. Your role is that of an observer, not consciously directing your breathing.

Open your eyes halfway, so that your eyelids block the upper half of your field of vision. Feel as if you are looking downward into your body, observing your posture and the sensation of breathing. Your gaze is soft, not focused tightly on a spot. Tune in to the sensation of your breathing, the feeling that your torso is filling with air as you breathe in and then emptying as you breathe out.

The practice of mindful awareness includes training yourself in returning to the present moment. At some point your mind will wander into a series of thoughts, away from attention on your posture and the sensation of your breathing. When you realize your mind is someplace else, just think, "Back to here and now," and return to focus on your posture and breathing, without judging or criticizing yourself for wandering.

Mindful Awareness of Sense Perceptions

Once you are settled, you can use mindful awareness to connect to the present moment by shifting your focus from one particular sense perception to another—seeing, hearing, feeling. Just notice as much as you can, with no need for mental commentary.

With eyes open, soften your gaze to expand your field vision in all directions. Let visual details fill your awareness, without moving your eyes. Notice shapes, colors, and shades of light and dark. Then, with eyes still open, turn your attention to sounds—near and far, loud and soft, from all directions. Notice that when you are focusing on sounds, you hear things you didn't when you were focusing on vision. Finally, still keeping your eyes open, turn your attention to bodily sensations—the weight of your body on the chair; the texture of your clothes against your skin; your torso moving with your breath; and your heartbeat or pulse. Since sense perceptions only occur in the present, this practice helps you experience staying in the present moment longer than you might have thought possible.

Then relax into an open mind, waiting for a thought. Notice how a thought suddenly appears as if from nowhere, lingers for a moment, and then disappears. Then simply be open to the next thought. Let thoughts come and go across your mind, like birds flying across the sky. In the tradition of mindful awareness, the mental recognition of thoughts is just another sense perception.

You will discover that when one sense is in the foreground of your awareness, all the others move to the background.

Environmental Awareness

Having practiced grounding, close placement, and mindful awareness of sense perceptions, a further component of training the mind is developing environmental awareness, a more panoramic perspective. In this practice your eyes are again fully open and your gaze is softened. As your breath moves out into the space in front of you, let your mind be open to the environment around you. Your mind can move to different objects of attention—sights, sounds, smells, thoughts, and feelings—as long as they are in the here and now.

If your mind wanders into a series of thoughts, when you realize your mind is someplace else, just think, "Back to here and now," and return to focus on your posture, breathing, and environment, without judging or criticizing yourself for getting distracted.

Continue the practice of opening out and resting in spaciousness with each outbreath. In that way, you begin to get a wider perspective on your thought process. You can experience thoughts and other sense perceptions clearly and distinctly as they arise.

In this practice the difference between being awake and daydreaming is very noticeable. When your mind is in the past, in the future, or wandering somewhere else in the present, you're not awake to your immediate environment. You're off in a daydream, asleep to the direct experience of the here and now. The ideal state of mind is to be as awake as you can be.

Don't get discouraged if you find your mind wandering a lot.

You can't force yourself to stay in the present. Continue the practice of returning, without judgment, to the object of your attention in the here and now. Eventually your mind will settle down.

Expansive Awareness

The final stage of a mind training session is expanding your awareness infinitely in all directions. It is an extension of the environmental awareness practice. With a very soft gaze, looking straight ahead, rest in awareness of the environment around you. With each successive outbreath, expand the scope of your awareness in stages. Imagine that your awareness opens out to the horizon, then to the sky, and then beyond the sky into space. Finally, imagine that your awareness extends in all directions farther than the farthest star, and rest in that infinite openness for as long as you can.

In that state you are completely open, your mind is limitless, and at the same time you are as centered as you can be.

Closing the Practice

Traditionally, each session of mindful awareness practice closes with an aspiration. If you choose to, in your own words you can say that you will be as mindfully aware as possible throughout the rest of the day or evening. You can also make the aspiration that training your mind will not only make you better at dieting, but a more genuine and decent human being, able to connect in a direct and helpful way with others.

ACKNOWLEDGMENTS

There are many people to whom I am grateful for their contribution to the development of this book. Whatever wisdom may be expressed in this work is what I learned from my teachers, Venerable Vidyadhara Chögyam Trungpa Rinpoche, Vajra Regent Ösel Tendzin, and Venerable Khenchen Thrangu Rinpoche. They have shown what it means to live in the present with unconditional confidence, wisdom, kindness, and compassion. Appreciation to many other great masters and practitioners of meditation with whom I have had the privilege of studying, including my long-time friend Pema Chödrön.

Special thanks to my contributing author/editors: my friend, Ken Zeiger, and my sister, Nancy Parent, for their invaluable contributions to make this book the best it can be. The beautiful cover is the work of my beautiful wife, Megan. Appreciation to readers who offered many helpful comments, including Megan, her daughter Caitlin Youngquist, Ladye Eugenia Stewart, and Dr. Caitlin Matthews.

Thanks to many dear friends who have supported and encouraged my work over the years: Ed Hanczaryk, Lyle Weinstein, Edward and Valerie Sampson, Glen Kakol, Lila Rich, Avilda Moses, Randy Sunday, Angela Rinaldi, Ryan Judkins, Gavin Lee, Mark Mushkin, Mark Moore, Chris Higgins, Joy and Eric Stephenson-Laws, Mike Donohue, Ken and Betty Potalivo, Mark and Nina Montoya, Ray and Sue Carrasco, and many more.

Thanks to the friends who have been willing to lend their celebrity to help increase awareness of my teaching, including Michael Bolton, Rick Dees, Cristie Kerr, Vijay Singh, Malcolm McDowell, George Lopez, Anthony Anderson, Mark Frost, Robby Krieger, Bill Scanlon, Ernie Els, Patrick Warburton, Michael O'Keefe, Kevin James, Ray Romano, and many others.

Last but not least, deep gratitude to my wife Megan and my whole family for their encouragement in my work on this book. Mom, my sister Nancy and her husband Michael, my brother Jack and his wife Kelly, and many dear cousins, have all been tremendously supportive and encouraging of my teaching and writing.

Whatever has not been presented clearly in this book is my responsibility alone. Any insights or benefit that have come from this work are due solely to the kindness of my teachers.

REFERENCES AND RECOMMENDED READINGS

Bays, Jan Chozen. *Mindful Eating.* Boston: Shambhala, 2009.

Beck, Charlotte Joko. *Everyday Zen.* New York: HarperCollins, 1989.

Chödrön, Pema. *Start Where You Are.* Boston: Shambhala, 1994.

Chödrön, Pema. *When Things Fall Apart.* Boston: Shambhala, 1997.

Chödrön, Pema. *The Places That Scare You.* Boston: Shambhala, 2001.

Frankl, Viktor. *Man's Search for Meaning.* Boston: Beacon Press, 1959.

Glasser, William. *Reality Therapy.* New York: Harper Paperbacks, 1989.

Hahn, Thich Nhat. *The Miracle of Mindfulness.*

   Boston: Beacon Press, 1975.

Hahn, Thich Nhat. *Peace is Every Step.* New York: Bantam, 1991.

Hahn, Thich Nhat. *Savor: Mindful Eating, Mindful Life.*

   New York: HarperCollins, 2010.

Kabat-Zinn, Jon. *Wherever You Go, There You Are.*

   New York: Hyperion, 1994.

Leonard, George. *Mastery.* New York: Dutton Plume, 1992.

Milne, A. A. *Winnie the Pooh.* Boston: E.P. Dutton, 1926.

Parent, Joseph. *Zen Golf: Mastering the Mental Game.*

   New York: Doubleday, 2002.

Parent, Joseph and Scanlon, Bill. *Zen Tennis: Playing in the Zone.*

   Ojai: Zen Arts, 2015.

Reps, Paul and Nyogen Senzaki. *Zen Flesh, Zen Bones.*

   Boston: Tuttle Publishing, 1957.

Suzuki, Shunryu. *Zen Mind, Beginner's Mind.*

   New York: Weatherhill, 1970.

Tendzin, Ösel. *Buddha in the Palm of Your Hand.*
Boston: Shambhala, 1982.

Tendzin, Ösel. *Chariot of Liberation.* Halifax: Vajradhatu, 2002.

Tendzin, Ösel. *Space, Time and Energy.* Ojai: Satdharma, 2004.

Trungpa, Chögyam. *Shambhala: The Sacred Path of the Warrior.*
Boston: Shambhala, 1984.

Trungpa, Chögyam. *Great Eastern Sun.* Boston: Shambhala, 1999.

Walton, Alice. "The 6 Weight-Loss Tips That Science Actually Knows
Work." Forbes Media, September 4, 2013.

Wansink, Brian. *Mindless Eating.* New York: Bantam, 2006.

Wansink, Brian. *Slim by Design.* New York: Bantam, 2014.

Williamson, Marianne. *A Course in Weight Loss.*
Carlsbad: Hay House, 2012.

Yeshe, Lama Thubten. *When the Chocolate Runs Out.*
Somerville: Wisdom, 2011.

ABOUT THE AUTHOR

DR. JOSEPH PARENT is a highly regarded author, speaker, and coach of Performance Psychology for wellness, business, and sports. He received his under-graduate degree from Cornell University and his Ph.D. from the University of Colorado. He has studied, practiced and taught mindful awareness and principles of psychology and communication in the Buddhist tradition since the 1970's in the lineage of Ven. Chögyam Trungpa, one of the great teachers to come to the West from Tibet.

Dr. Parent is the best-selling author of *ZEN GOLF: Mastering the Mental Game*, with a million copies in print, digital, and audio formats worldwide, as well as several other books. He is available for coaching in wellness, business and sports by voice or video calls anywhere in the world.

Dr. Parent has spoken at numerous conferences, meetings, management retreats and training programs for a wide variety of businesses and associations. He offers Mindful Awareness training, corporate seminars and executive coaching, as well as sports psychology lessons. He teaches in person at the Ojai Valley Inn and Spa resort in Ojai, California, where he makes his home with his wife, Megan.

ZEN AND THE ART OF
WELLNESS, BUSINESS, AND SPORTS
WITH
DR. JOE PARENT

Keynote Speaking
Executive Coaching
Corporate Mindfulness Programs
Business and Sports Events
Private Lessons

Dr. Parent is based at the spectacular
Ojai Valley Inn and Spa,
a world-renowned resort in the
magical Ojai Valley of Southern California.

For information on Dr. Parent's speaking and coaching, in person and by voice or video calls anywhere in the world, as well as his audio, video, and on-line instructional materials, please visit: thebestdietbookever.com or zengolf.com

DrJoe@thebestdietbookever.com
805.640.1046

Made in the USA
Coppell, TX
16 September 2024